WILD ADVENTURES WITH YOUR CANINE FRIEND

BY ANGELA JONES

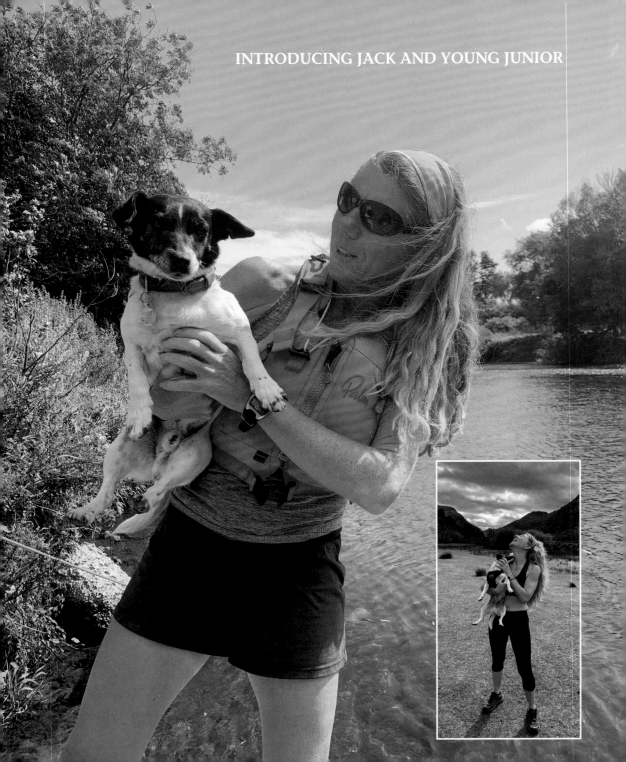

HELLO

I am Angela Jones and for 57 years on this beautiful planet, I've lived a life without lanes.

Sharing this joy over the last 14 years has been my constant companion Jack – my rescue dog and co-adventurer.

I want to share my love and knowledge of our wonderful adventures together, how we grew as a team, Jack's training progression, safety tips and some of our exciting travel adventures together.

The great outdoors has so much to share and is available to all. We can all enjoy the same health and wellbeing benefits that compliment us and our canine friends, but all the time we must respect and protect nature.

Exciting, fun, wild adventure runs through our hearts, veins and our 6 paws! I am fortunate to have shared many wild remote and extreme wild adventures with my woofs over the years. I've had a lifetime of wild swimming, kayaking and wild camping, trail running and paddle boarding on the River Wye and way beyond, while always appreciating and respecting Nature's beauty and diversity.

The Wye river is my office and playground and where Jack and I have run our Adventure Business for over a decade. www.angelajoneswimwild.co.uk

We have been recognised and presented with many Adventure and Environmental Awards over the years. My business has never been about expansion, but about sharing my vast knowledge and respect of the great outdoors to enhance others' confidence and wellbeing as well as being inclusive to our canine friends.

I have written this book to share my life-long passion of adventure and the sheer joy that my beloved Jack Russells brought to it. And how you too can introduce your best friend to safe and healthy adventures together, whatever their breed and ability.

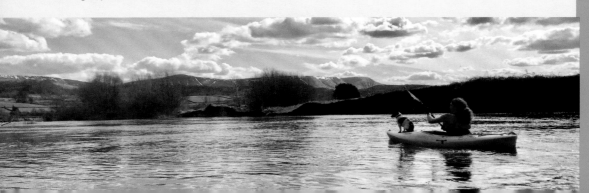

"WILD ADVENTURES WITH YOUR CANINE FRIEND"

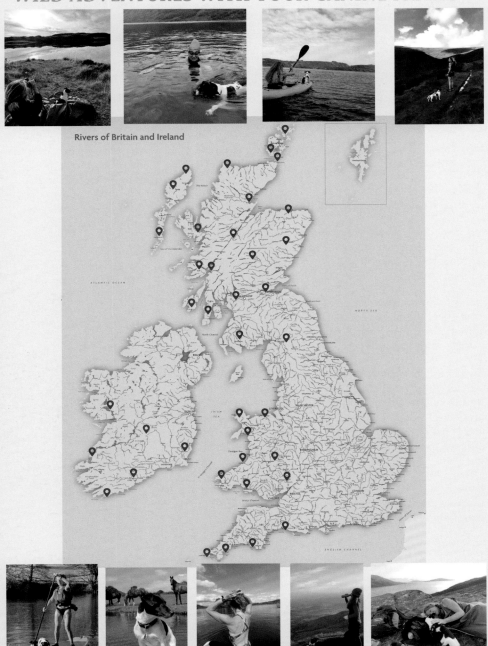

Rivers of Britain and Ireland

Some of our recent adventure areas

Contents

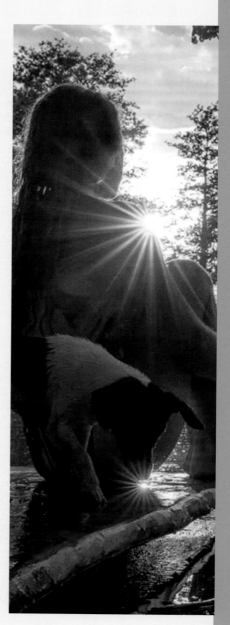

Image: G Katewood

A bit more about the author and Jack

Me? Well, I'm a rather feral person and a life-long wild swimmer, kayaker, trail runner and wild camper. My life has been full of spontaneity and adventure, with plenty of challenging aspects along the way, to say the least. I live in the moment - the here and now.

My energy and enthusiasm for Nature and the great outdoors oozes out of every pore of my weather-hardened skin. I do not over-analyse, I don't stress, I don't hold onto negatives – I just live in the moment.

I was born in Greenford and moved several times before leaving home at 15. I grew up fast and tough. I remember a careers officer in school asking what I wanted to do when I left. I replied, "Have a life of adventure and exploring." Where or what, I didn't know.

After many years of travelling and exploring, I settled and continued my adventurous life with my children in the Welsh hills. The day Jack entered my life was a very strange

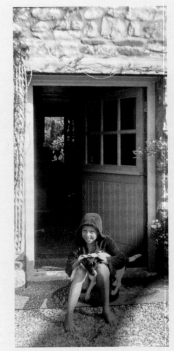

Jack is welcomed to our farm by my son

one. I lived on a farm in the countryside, which was stunningly peaceful. I was the worst farmer possible as every animal we had became a pet. After renovating a run-down barn and living in a caravan for 2 years, the barn finally became our home where my young children ran free and shared the fields with sheep, emus, ducks, chickens and the odd goat.

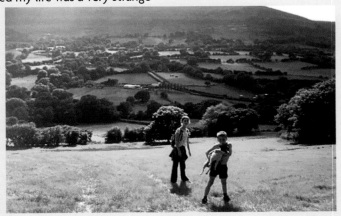

Jack joins us on our family farm with fields of gold

Life has a way of shaking you up and after three burglaries in a matter of weeks the decision was made to get a yappy dog to warn us of strangers.

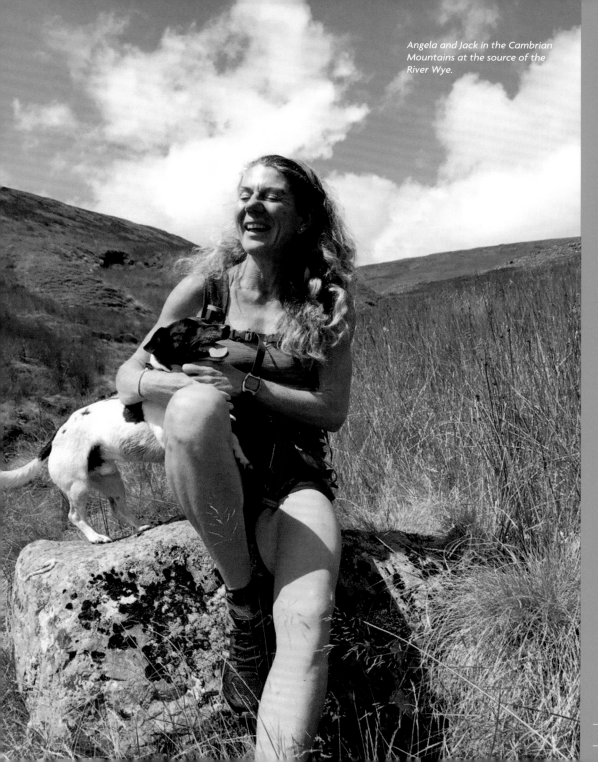

Angela and Jack in the Cambrian Mountains at the source of the River Wye.

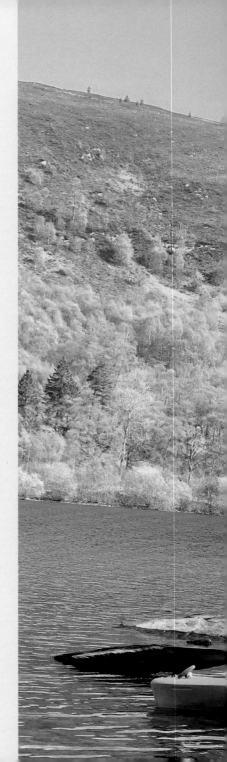

Jack came into my life suddenly and in a totally unexpected way. He was about a year old and had been treated badly; he was very nervous and would often roll onto his back and wet himself. He didn't like loud noises or men with bald heads, but what I do remember was he loved laughter and children. He took a while to settle into the freedom and fun of farm life and the fields and rivers of gold in Wales, but soon become a huge essential part of our crazy adventurous lives.

I remember when we first cycled together. He ran by my side along the canal and he caught a squirrel, which I ended up bringing home in my top and putting by the fire to warm and revive. Jack had his first lesson about not chasing wildlife – I didn't need words, he just knew instinctively that what he had done had caused harm to wildlife and that wasn't part of what my whole ethos is about.

Yes, he is a terrier and you may say 'a rabbiter', and yes, it's 'in their blood' but like humans, dogs can also adapt and learn respect for each other and their surroundings. The day he first got to see me kayaking, watching from the garden on the canal, he didn't have a clue what was happening. He just followed close by my side observing and thinking, "What is this crazy lady doing?" Funny to think for the next 14 years this would be his norm and his passion too.

When I slipped into the local river for a swim on one of his first walks he just sat and watched. Jack soon caught onto my thinking and became the most amazing kind, chilled dog there was. Little did he know that the bond we would build and the life ahead would be totally amazing.

A dog is intuitive. They will pick up on what your aura is all about and how you see the world. Stress feeds stress. Jack quickly became part of the family and grew used to the fun adventures we all had.

I remember the first time I took Jack on a longer run in the hills and he wouldn't even put his paw in the stream to cross it. I patiently let him work it out for himself and never fussed over him. My life is pretty basic. I have no set routines, no planning, no over-thinking, and never ever stress. My connection and respect for Nature comes naturally and never has to be thought about.

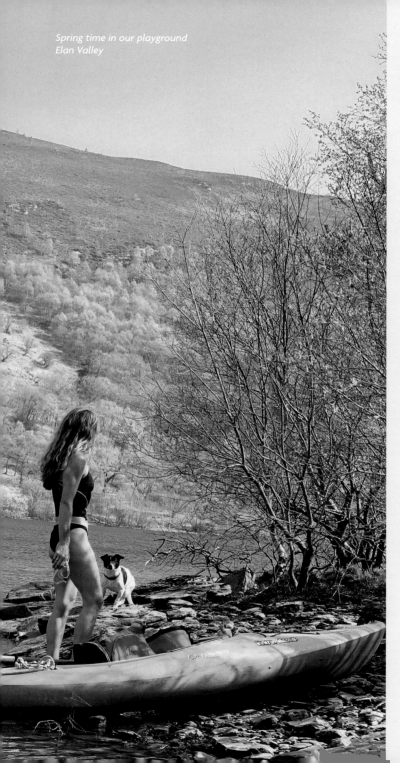

Spring time in our playground
Elan Valley

One of my great loves is sharing Nature – watching, absorbing and being part of the circle that forms a connection without words.

Jack had a big job on his hands to understand that life was not about being owned or being told what to do, but instead to use his imagination and intuition, simply to be himself. Jack, and I and you, are all unique and individual, so why would we want to be on a lead? As long as I set some ground rules and shared safety aspects his life, like mine, would be pretty spontaneous and wild, with a huge amount of fun and enjoyment thrown in.

As my children grew and fled the nest Jack became part of a primarily wild, feral, and wonderful life.

My office and playground was, and still is, the great outdoors and so many wondrous wild adventures were about to follow.

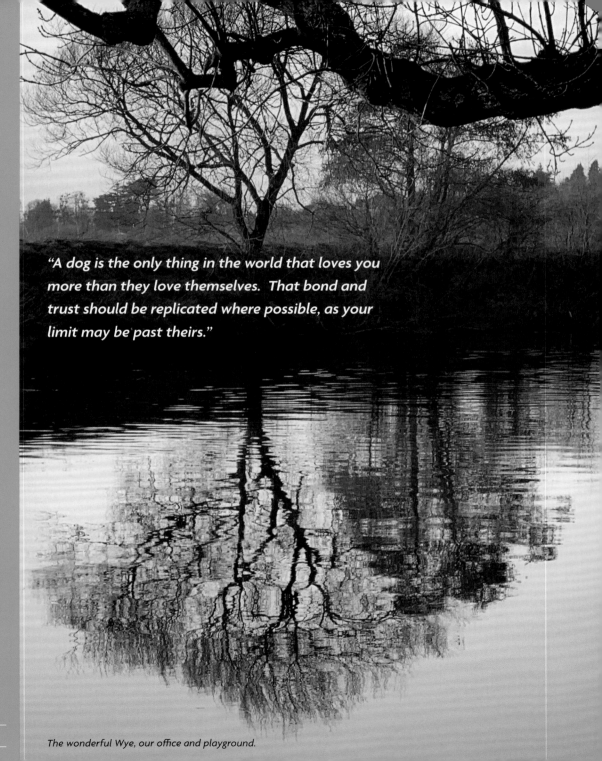

"*A dog is the only thing in the world that loves you more than they love themselves. That bond and trust should be replicated where possible, as your limit may be past theirs.*"

The wonderful Wye, our office and playground.

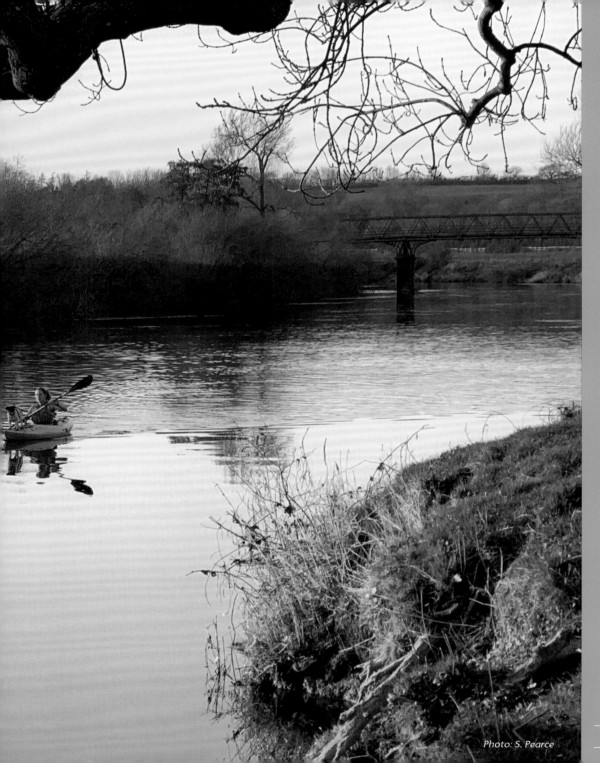

Photo: S. Pearce

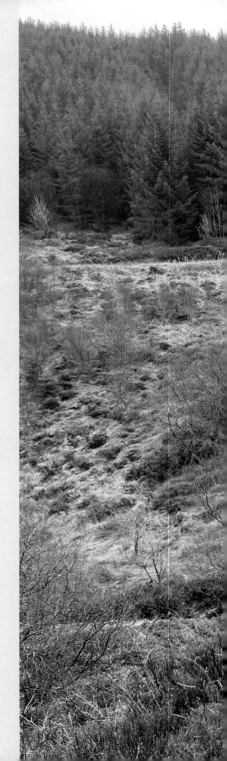

To avoid fatigue; make sure your dog is healthy before you attempt any adventure

If you've ever started a workout routine from a fitness level of, let's say 'zero', you know that it's tough going.

The road to peak performance takes time. And while you may be more than ready to get back to the active lifestyle that's been on pause for the past couple of years, if your dog is your hiking, running, swimming, or kayaking buddy they may need some time to increase their own fitness levels and build up their endurance too.

Remember that your dog will always want to please, so will exhaust itself to keep up with you!

Paw pads need time to develop the calluses that will protect their feet on rougher terrain. It's always best to do moderate, controlled outdoor adventures first and then build up gradually.

When in doubt, please ask a vet.
Anytime you have a change in lifestyle that involves your dog, it's wise to have them checked over by your vet. Maybe this is the summer you take up camping, trail running, kayaking etc. and these new adventures could mean new experiences for your dog. Your vet will be able to take this information and make any necessary adjustments to your dog's vaccines, parasite control, or other proactive healthcare recommendations. Prevention is better than cure.

Puppies develop much faster than children, so the first year is critical.

1. Make sure your dog has a clean bill of health
2. Work gradually on improving fitness levels
3. Ensure your dog is up to date with all necessary jabs
4. Work on trust, boundaries, rules and commands
5. Remember that a dog is a pack animal and you need to be the head of that pack when it comes to leadership.

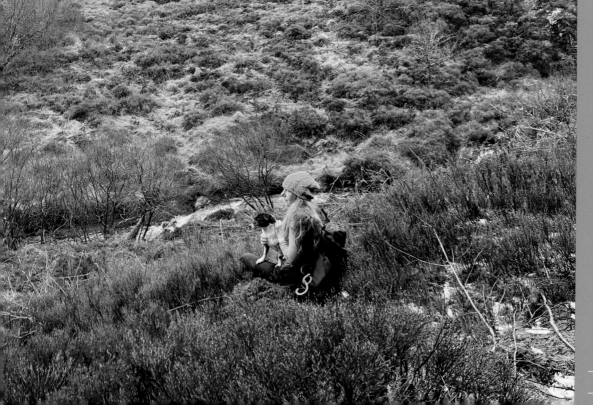

DOG TO HUMAN AGE COMPARISONS	
PUPPY	**HUMAN**
0-3 weeks: eyes, ears open	0-1 year
6 weeks: playful, more co-ordinated	2 years
8 weeks: ready to go to new home	3 years
12 weeks	4 years
16 weeks	6 years
24 weeks: puberty	8 years
8 months	14 years
12 months: beginning of adulthood	20 years
18 months: social maturity	24 years
7 years: middle age	50 years
10 years: onset of old age	70 years
15 years	90 years

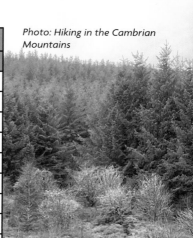

Photo: Hiking in the Cambrian Mountains

Teach your pup to respect wildlife

Larry was an orphaned lamb and he and Jack were buddies for years.

Jack always generously shared food with all his wild friends.

You can't teach an old dog new tricks but you can certainly mentor the 'new pup on the block'. Wise and wild aspects of respect. Teach your dog to respect wildlife from a pup.

My Jack learned to enjoy and embrace wildlife and Nature and would often nurse orphaned and injured animals. This lamb, Larry, was orphaned and grew up with Jack as best friends. Jack also played 'big brother' to the odd rabbit, a seagull, ducklings, chickens and even emus over the years. We would often sit still for hours and just watch and admire wildlife at close quarters. Never a bark or a stir was made, as this was part of the magic that Jack and I had with Nature.

We knew all the quiet magical places along the river and woods. We would watch the vixen come out with her cubs night after night; we knew where the deer came to drink as the sun set below the cliffs of the Wye; we knew where the swans would congregate in the summer months – the one with the crooked neck would always mesmerise us.

Jack would swim with me for hours, playing and watching the ripples of the fish merge as they sometimes jumped to the surface. We would watch the heron devouring a fish – enjoying his tea. We watched kingfishers dive, minnows nibble my feet, and we got so familiar with the otters in their holts that they trusted us enough to let their two pups join us one day in the river. The mother gave a little but strict squeal to tell them to come back.

Jack loved the excitement of watching and discovering many wonderful animals and so much beautiful wildlife during his 15-year life.

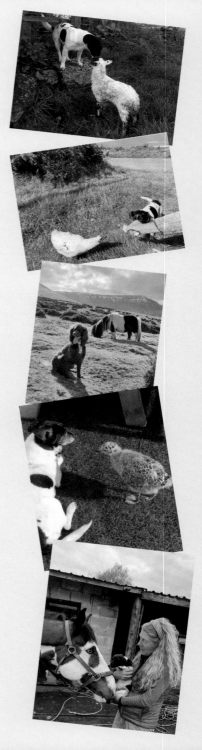

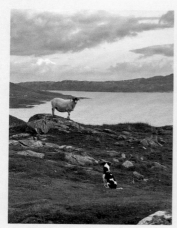

Curiosity in the Outer Hebrides

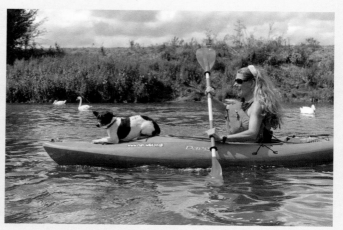

Many people think it's inherent in a breed to chase or attack wildlife but I feel a dog will always embrace, enjoy and respect wildlife like its guardian when led to understand the beauty in everything wild.

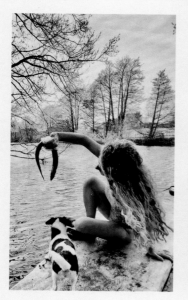

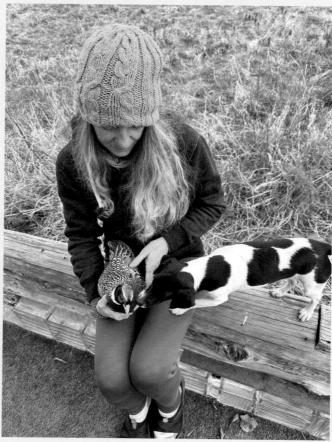

Junior and I nurse a pheasant back to health

WILD SWIMMING WITH YOUR DOG

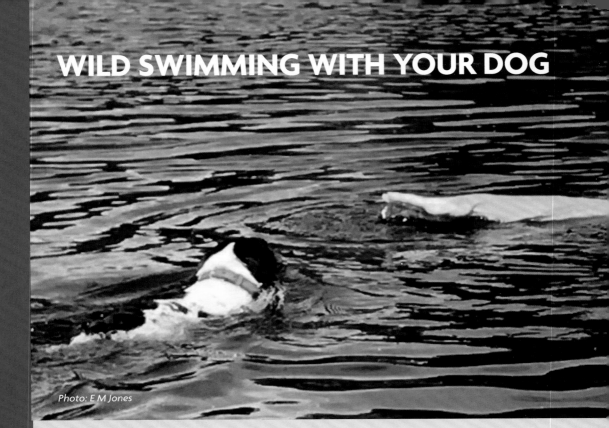

Photo: E M Jones

I will cheerfully share with you my decades of knowledge on how to prepare your pup/dog for the water, the best practices for canine water safety, and mention some water-related medical issues to look out for. Whether it's time spent walking along the river bank, or actually in the water kayaking or wild swimming with your dog, it is extremely important that you know your water safety capabilities at all your favourite rivers, lakes, streams and beaches.

Your dog trusts you and loves you and will put their life in your hands. Remember that whatever adventure you are on, it is your idea and you have big responsibilities for your four-legged friend.

A responsible owner is a capable and informed owner, so be well prepared and keep you and your 'water dog' safe with these tips.

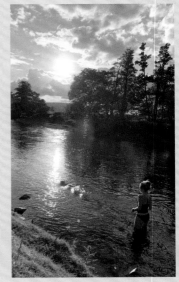

Evening swim in the Usk River

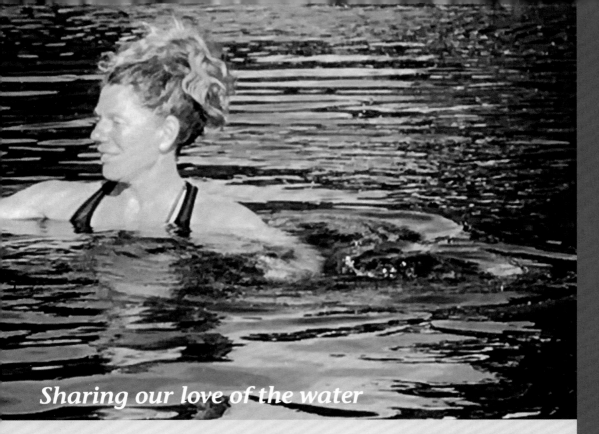

Sharing our love of the water

Prepare your woof for the water

Whilst it's easy to assume that all dogs love the water and are "natural-born swimmers," that's not always the case. Some don't like the water but all dogs need to learn to swim for their own safety. Give your dog time to acclimatise slowly by playing – throwing a safe stick or ball into the shallow water is a good way to start.

Never hurry them to swim. Let them adjust and learn in their own time, otherwise you could put them off all together. Sadly, I can tell you that over the years I've watched too many pet owners distress their dog by forcing the situation to meet their own means. Water should be fun and also needs to be respected. If your dog sees you embracing and enjoying it naturally, then they will trust that it is an adventurous fun thing to share.

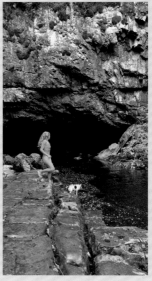

Brecon Beacons

Remember, just as with humans, fear and fatigue can overwhelm canine swimmers of any level, so carefully monitor your dog around the water. Dog life jackets are a great idea if you and your dog plan to spend time on or near the water, especially if kayaking, paddle boarding or canoeing. These flotation devices are a great safety precaution but often require some getting used to. Always get your dog accustomed to it on dry land first.

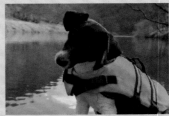

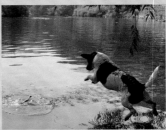

Jack's favourite thing was to dive into water from the bank and ledges, but just like with humans, you need to make sure you've fully assessed the area and entry point of the water. Always take the time to find a safe swimming area. Even though it was Jack's favourite thing, as a result of training and trust he would always wait for me to assess the area (even if it was a familiar spot – things can change) and to say, "Go" before he leapt into the water.

Jack would always wait for the command before entering the water.

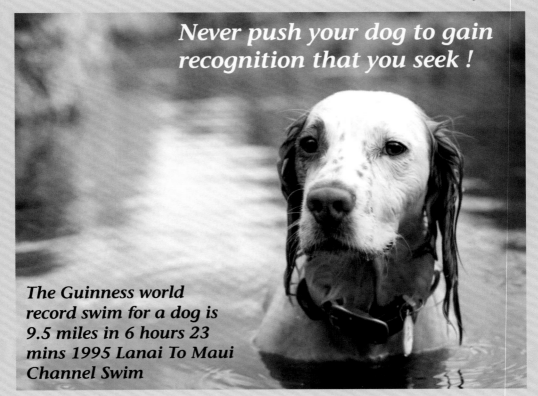

Never push your dog to gain recognition that you seek !

The Guinness world record swim for a dog is 9.5 miles in 6 hours 23 mins 1995 Lanai To Maui Channel Swim

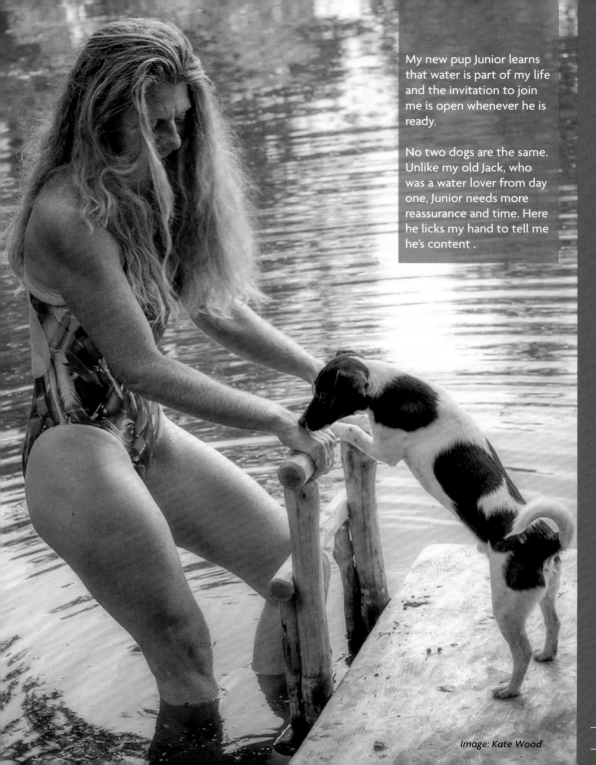

My new pup Junior learns that water is part of my life and the invitation to join me is open whenever he is ready.

No two dogs are the same. Unlike my old Jack, who was a water lover from day one, Junior needs more reassurance and time. Here he licks my hand to tell me he's content .

Image: Kate Wood

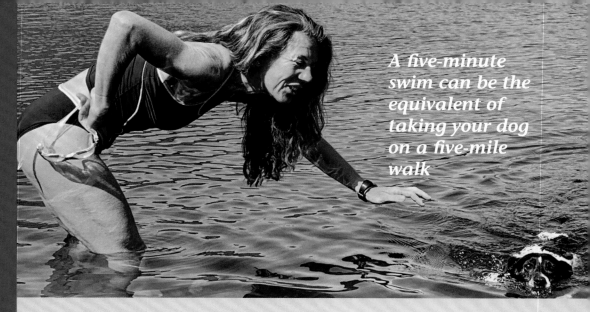

A five-minute swim can be the equivalent of taking your dog on a five-mile walk

Teaching Your Dog To Swim

If you go to a popular doggy swimming area you are sure to see loads of happy dogs enjoying a good splash about in the water. Most dogs absolutely love water and many are naturally very strong swimmers. However, not all dog breeds are confident swimmers or they may have had a bad experience in the water. If you can encourage your dog to swim, it is wonderful form of exercise. It is said that a five-minute swim can be the equivalent of taking your dog on a five-mile walk.

Don't bother trying to get a Bulldog to swim – his small legs won't keep him afloat and he won't survive long as a submarine.

It can be tempting to encourage your dog to swim when the weather is warm. But be mindful that even if they look lovely, some places can be unsafe and might have strong currents that can be dangerous. High algae and bacteria levels can also make your dog sick.

Instead, try to find clear, clean shallow streams which your dog can just paddle in briefly to cool off. Always ensure you provide them with separate clean water in a water bowl for

them to drink and take your walks at the coolest parts of the day.

If you think that your dog is losing fitness or becoming overweight, swimming is a great way to burn calories. It is an effective way of increasing your dog's strength and flexibility, whilst lowering his body fat at the same time. Always take a towel with you to dry off your dog before taking them home. And if possible, rinse your dog off with fresh water after they have had a swim to get rid of any chemicals or algae. You can buy little portable 'dog showers' to carry in the car.

How To Teach Your Dog To Swim

Confidence is the key, so it is important that you start off slowly. Allow your dog to become comfortable with getting wet by walking them into the water on the lead. You might have to persuade them with a couple of treats or their favourite toy, but make sure that you reassure your dog with a positive voice and lots of praise. After a few minutes you can start to venture into deeper water so that they have to begin paddling to stay afloat.

At this point you might need to support their tummy with one hand if you notice them sinking. If your dog starts to panic, bring it into the shallow water so that it can calm down and regain confidence, and then try again. Treat your dog when they get out and shake themself off so that they can relate swimming to a positive experience. They'll soon begin to love it.

Please remember that not all dogs like to swim, and forcing your dog to try isn't going to encourage a positive association with that activity. Let them take it slowly and get used to it at their own pace. Some days they simply may not feel like swimming. Even if a dog is a strong swimmer, they may not understand tides or currents, so it's important for you as their guardian, to assess any risks and keep your dog out of the water if the conditions are dangerous.

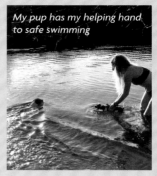

My pup has my helping hand to safe swimming

Whenever your dog is in an uncontrolled situation around water (like in a boat or canoe), make sure they are wearing a doggie life vest but definitely NOT a lead. Tragically, several pets have drowned when the kayak, paddle board or canoe has capsized and the dog has been attached by a lead and unable to free itself.

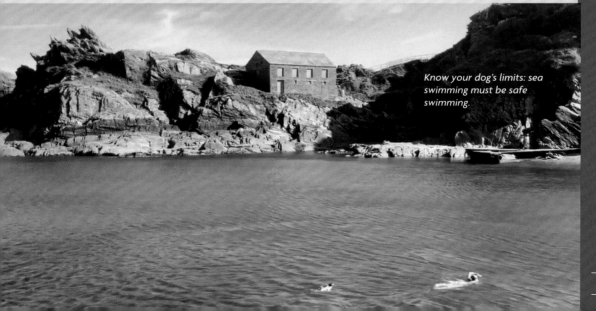

Know your dog's limits: sea swimming must be safe swimming.

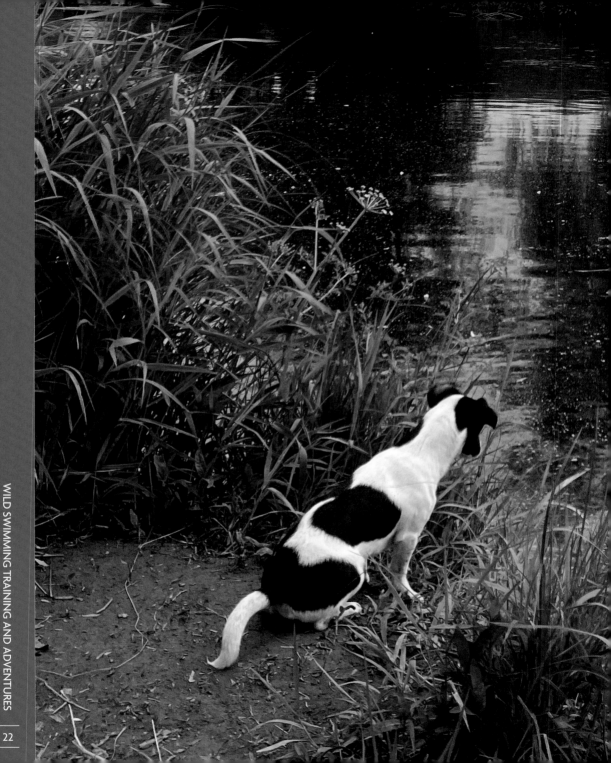

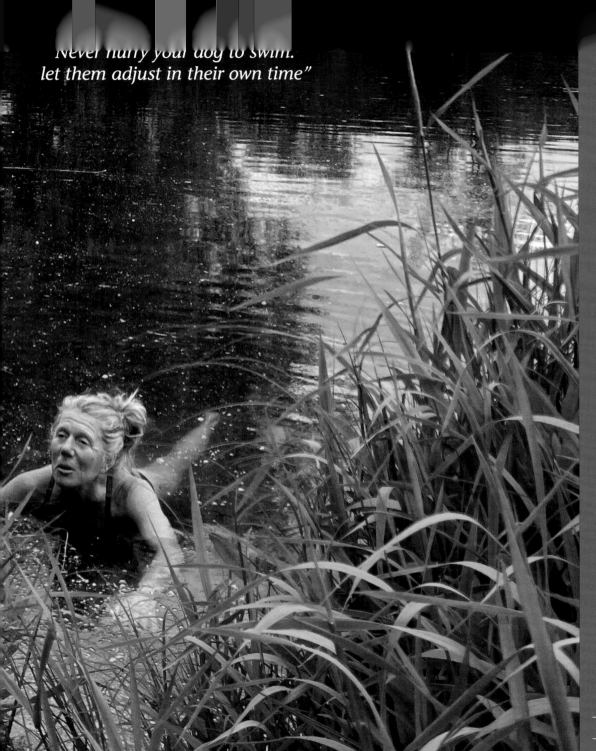

"Never hurry your dog to swim,
let them adjust in their own time"

Where can I teach my dog to swim?

Most importantly, make sure the water is clean. Over the years I've watched the horrendous decline in the 'wild water' quality, so am very choosey now and always test the sections regularly with my water testing kit. Sadly, some rivers, canals, lakes and reservoirs contain infectious diseases like Leptospirosis, so choose a spot that you know is safe and test the water if unsure. Never think it is safe just because other dogs swim there regularly. Learn to identify good water quality and harmful pollution *see pages 84-87*.

Never jump in to save a dog; they are more capable than you think.

Top ten safety tips

At Seas, Streams, Rivers and Lakes:
- Keep your dog out of water that you wouldn't swim in yourself. Beware of toxic algae blooms, submerged objects (on which a dog could be impaled), and areas guarded by aggressive wildlife.
- You'll have more peace of mind during "wild swimming" or boating activities if your dog's wearing a properly fitted, quality canine life jacket.
- Don't permit your dog to harass water fowl or local wildlife.
- Swimming can be more tiring than running, so watch for signs of fatigue, including trembling, heavy panting and/or swimming lower in the water or slower than usual.
- Continually monitor your dog In the rivers and oceans, where hazards are often multiplied.
- Don't encourage your dog to venture far from river banks or offshore. That means not throwing retriever toys and floats way out into the water. In the sea and rivers, your dog is vulnerable to rough currents, waves, riptides and cross-currents - all of which can be deadly.
- If your dog is a toy breed or has short legs or a short muzzle, consider outfitting them with a life jacket, whether or not they intentionally go into the water.
- Sea water is bad for dogs if ingested, so do your best to keep them from drinking it. Large amounts of saltwater can make your dog sick, and may even prove fatal. Offer them fresh drinking water regularly.

- Likewise, while your dog may love rolling in stinky fish and other things that wash up on the beach or river bank, they shouldn't eat them. Dead fish and other marine life can contain deadly toxins.
- Be aware of the sun and its strength. Over-exposure can be as hazardous to dogs as it is to humans. Seek shade throughout the day.

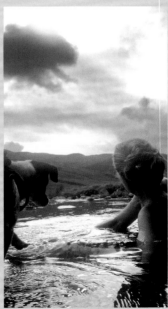

Embracing Highland Water after a long hiking day

Healthly swim tips

Keep your dog safe in open water whether it's a river, lake or sea. It is essential for us as pet guardians to know about water safety.

Water intoxication, also known as hyponatremia, can occur when dogs ingest large quantities of water very quickly. This can occur with dogs that repeatedly dive open-mouthed into the water to retrieve a ball or toy. It's relatively rare but potentially fatal. Excessive water in the system causes electrolyte levels to drop, thinning blood plasma, leading to swelling of the brain and other organs.

"Swimmer's tail," or Acute Caudal Myopathy (aka limber-tail syndrome), typically affects large-breed dogs, causing the dog's tail to droop after too much time playing in the water.

This type of over-exertion can strain the muscles that keep a dog's tail up and wagging. Along with tail limpness, the base of the tail is often stiff, and the dog may experience pain.

A 10-minute swim is equivalent to a 40-minute run for your dog so <u>your</u> limit may be past <u>their</u> limit !!!

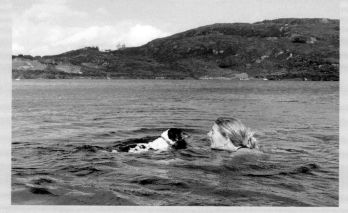

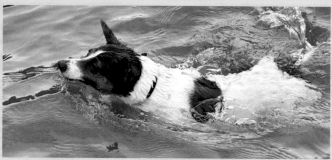

High back and tail shows good swim position and energetic dog, and as the dog tires the back and tail drop.

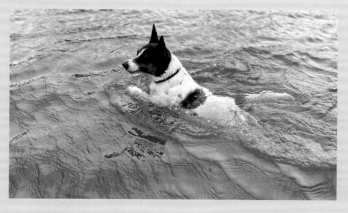

Always keep an eye on the tail and spine as they will start to drop lower as dog tires.

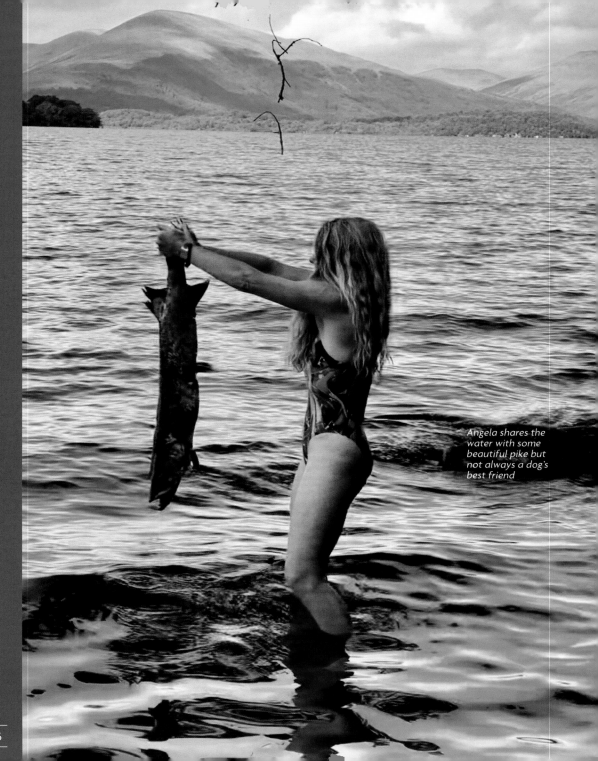

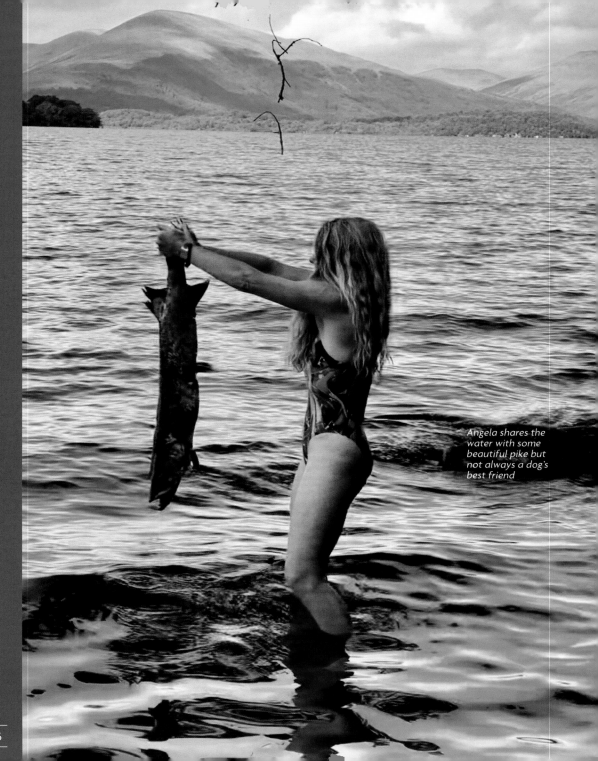Angela shares the water with some beautiful pike but not always a dog's best friend

Fishing Dangers

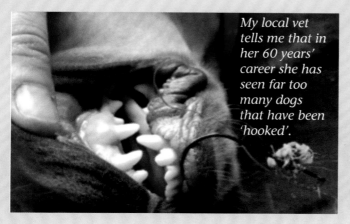

My local vet tells me that in her 60 years' career she has seen far too many dogs that have been 'hooked'.

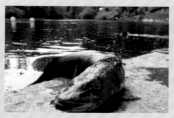

Decaying fish can be harmful to dogs if ingested

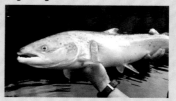

Beware of fishhooks. If your dog is swimming, kayaking, paddle boarding with you whilst others are fishing, or in an area where people fish, always be alert. Keep your dog away from tackle boxes and whatever fish may have been caught to prevent them from swallowing fishhooks.

And of course, don't allow your dog to get accidentally hooked. Keep them at a safe distance away from casting lines. When you are in and on the river or any water source, you need to be vigilant for both of you.

On the subject of fish – salmon-type fish (salmon, trout, char and others) found in our rIvers and coasts can carry a parasitic fluke (a type of worm) infected with a micro-organism called Neorickettsia helminthoeca. Dogs who eat these fish raw may come down with salmon poisoning disease (SPD), symptoms of which include fever, enlarged lymph nodes, and debilitating

diarrhoea and vomiting. Left untreated, SPD is fatal to 90% of the dogs that contract it. Contact your vet immediately if you think your dog has ingested any of these fish.

A study has revealed that, highly toxic insecticides used on dogs to kill fleas and ticks are poisoning rivers across the UK. This discovery is 'extremely concerning' for water insects, and the fish and birds that depend on them. Scientists have warned that 'significant environmental damage is being done'.

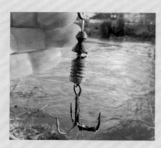

Increased litter discarded by anglers in Britain is having a devastating affect on domestic animals and wildlife. I'm constantly finding hooks and lines. A true fisherman respects Nature.

My local vet tells me that in her 60 years' career she has seen far too many dogs that have been 'hooked'.

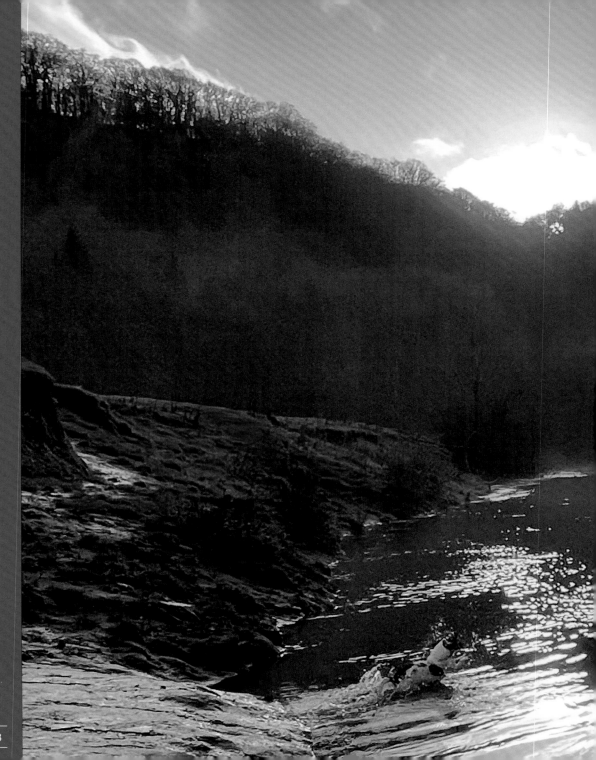

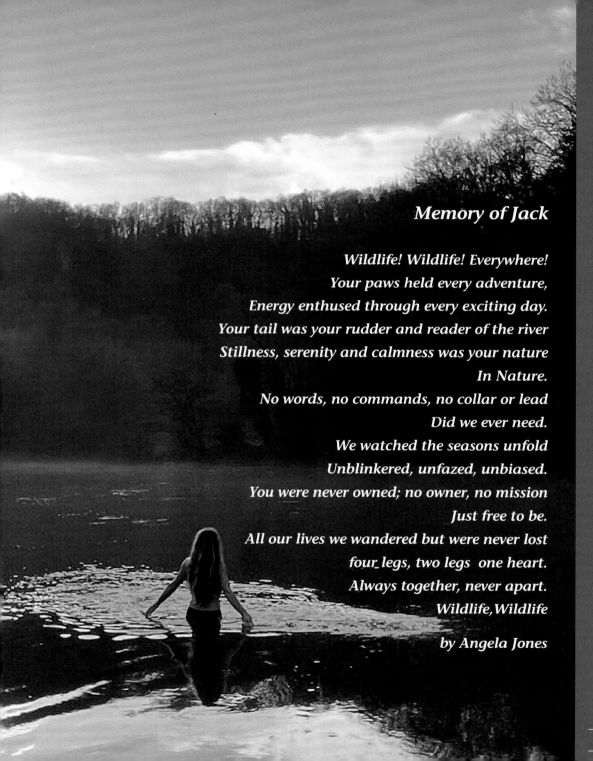

Memory of Jack

Wildlife! Wildlife! Everywhere!
Your paws held every adventure,
Energy enthused through every exciting day.
Your tail was your rudder and reader of the river
Stillness, serenity and calmness was your nature
In Nature.
No words, no commands, no collar or lead
Did we ever need.
We watched the seasons unfold
Unblinkered, unfazed, unbiased.
You were never owned; no owner, no mission
Just free to be.
All our lives we wandered but were never lost
four legs, two legs one heart.
Always together, never apart.
Wildlife, Wildlife

by Angela Jones

SUMMER ADVENTURE RISKS WITH YOUR DOG

Avoiding heatstroke and dehydration

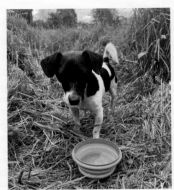

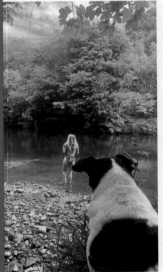

The photo pictured left shows Jack chilling in the shade as I go for a midday swim. Our swims together changed to early morning or late evenings in the height of summer.

Keeping your dog cool in hot weather is all about being prepared and thinking ahead. As well as having fun when the weather gets warmer it's important to think about keeping your dog safe in the heat. The aim is to reduce the risk of heatstroke and make sure your dog stays healthy and happy. I've put together some top hot weather dog care tips, so you can enjoy the sun and keep your dog safe.

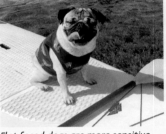

I always have fresh water and bowl for my dog

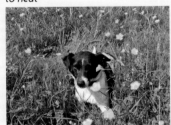

Flat faced dogs are more sensitive to heat

Plan your activities

Avoid adventures with your dog if the weather is hot as dogs are not able to cope in the heat as well as humans can. Even a warm day can cause dogs to overheat, especially if they're exercising. Your dog will be much safer going for a gentle adventure very early or late in the evening when the temperature has significantly reduced. Be mindful of the weather when planning activities and make sure you can take regular breaks in the shade.

ALWAYS REMEMBER TO CARRY WATER. Water availability is essential for your dog all year round, but especially on a hot day. If you're out and about with your dog, make sure you always have a bottle of water and a bowl for them to drink from.

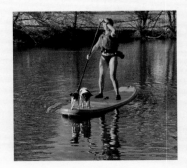

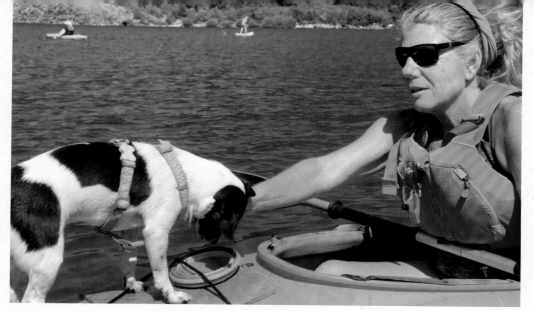

Junior gets a refreshing drink and keeps paws cool, on padded mat whilst summer kayaking in Snowdonia

Heatstroke and Dehydration

Just like people, dogs are at risk of heatstroke and dehydration when temperatures rise. How hot is too hot for your dog? If you're uncomfortable in the sun, your dog probably is too. Make sure your dog always has access to fresh water and shade when outside, even if just in the garden. Some dog breeds, such as Pugs, Bulldogs, Boston Terriers, and other flat-faced breeds, have a particularly tough time in hot weather. Their restricted airways put them at greater risk for heatstroke and make them less tolerant of exercise. Keep an extra close eye on them during warm days and let them be a couch potato if

they want to be. Please use common sense – you might want to go 'out to play on the water' but the priority must be your dog's health and well-being.

Summer also means the possibility of extra adventures like hiking, swimming, kayaking, paddle boarding and wild camping under the stars.

YOUR DOG IS NOT A TROPHY AND THERE TO SHOW HOW CLEVER THE OWNER IS – safety, enjoyment and sharing SAFE adventures is what it's all about.

Familiarise yourself with the signs of heatstroke

Dogs suffer with heatstroke when they overheat and can't reduce their body temperature. It can be fatal. Any dog can develop heatstroke, but overweight, young, elderly, flat-faced, giant-breed, and thick-coated dogs are particularly at risk, even from just sitting out in hot weather. This can happen not just when it's 'obviously hot' but also in warmer temperatures that often are 'assumed' to be safe. It is important to recognise and be aware of the signs of heatstroke at any stage, as it requires urgent veterinary treatment.

Signs of heatstroke include:

Heavy panting/Lethargy
Shaking or weakness
Confusion or loss of coordination
Seizures
Drooling or foaming at the mouth
Vomiting or diarrhoea

If you think your dog has heatstroke, you need to ACT FAST. Make sure you contact your vet immediately. Make sure you are familiar with these steps BEFORE you need to use them.

- Keep your dog calm and still.
- Put them on top of a cool wet towel, cooling mat, or place them in the breeze of a fan if possible.
- Allow the dog to drink small amounts of cool water.
- Pour cool water over the dog's feet, ears and head. Never use ice or very cold water as this can cause shock.
- Gradually start to move cool water over their body but not so much that they start shivering.
- If possible, continue cooling your dog on the way to your vet.

Protect paws

Surfaces that heat up in the sun, such as tarmac or sand, and even paddle boards, kayaks and canoes can be painful for your dog's paws. If in doubt, simply check for yourself. If it feels too hot for your 'paws', it will be too hot for your dog's paws too. Always stick to cool surfaces, like grass and if your activity includes paddling please check hard surfaces and choose cooler times of day to go out instead.

Adapt exercise

In warmer weather it's a good idea to find ways to stimulate your dog's mental and physical energy, which are less strenuous. For example, if they usually like to run for hours at a time this could be detrimental in hotter temperatures. Instead, you could hide their toys or treats in a small area and let them sniff them out, or you could

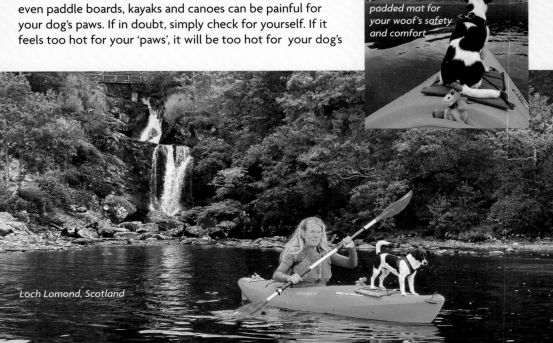

Overheated surface can burn paws so use padded mat for your woof's safety and comfort

Loch Lomond, Scotland

freeze their food or use frozen treats in toys, or food puzzle toys to keep them stimulated. Whatever activities you choose, make sure they are calm and out of the heat.

Never leave dogs in cars

Leaving a dog alone in a hot car can be fatal. Even if it is cool when you leave them, temperatures change very quickly and even in the shade with the windows open, the car interior can heat up enough to make dogs distressed and uncomfortable, which can lead to heatstroke very quickly. Make sure you always have a plan, so your dog isn't left alone in the car or any other enclosed spaces. If you see a distressed dog in a hot car, dial 999 immediately.

You should avoid travelling in your car with your dog on a hot day. If you do need to travel, make sure that you use shade covers on the windows, so they don't have direct sun on them whilst you are travelling. If possible cool your car down and have the air conditioning on before putting your dog in. Avoid travelling at hotter times of the day and consider travelling when there is less traffic, so you don't get stuck for long periods of time. Ensure your dog has access to water throughout the journey – there are some great non-splash bowls available on the market. Be prepared – you could be delayed or even break down – make sure you are able to take good care of your pet in such circumstances.

Keep your dog fit and healthy

It's important to help your dog stay as fit and healthy as possible all year round, whatever that might involve. Even during the wet winter months, when you may be inclined to spend less time outdoors, it's especially important to help them maintain a healthy weight. Your dog will likely be less active when it's cold and wet, so it can be a good idea to adjust the amount of food you give them to reflect how much energy they are using up. It's a great opportunity to practice basic tricks and training indoors where you keep up your relationship and help your dog's brain to remain active. Speak to your vet if you are concerned about your dog's weight or want advice on how to safely support your dog to lose weight. A healthy dog is better able to cope with all the different seasons and temperatures they bring.

Normal body temperature for dogs is from 101.0 to 102.5°F (38.3 to 39.2°C). Some people and some pets maintain a baseline temperature a little above or below the average. If your pet's temperature rises above 104°F (40.0°C) or falls below 99°F (37.2°C), take your pet to your vet immediately. Make sure you are familiar with what is normal for your dog.

Never leave your dog in a vehicle. All dog owners should know this, but it's always worth repeating. In warm weather, it can only take a matter of minutes for a dog to get heatstroke if left in a car unattended.

Only have pets in the car if you're in there with them, with the windows open or air conditioning on.

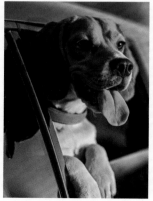

It takes minutes for a dog to get heatstroke in a car if unattended.

WINTER ADVENTURE RISKS WITH YOUR DOG

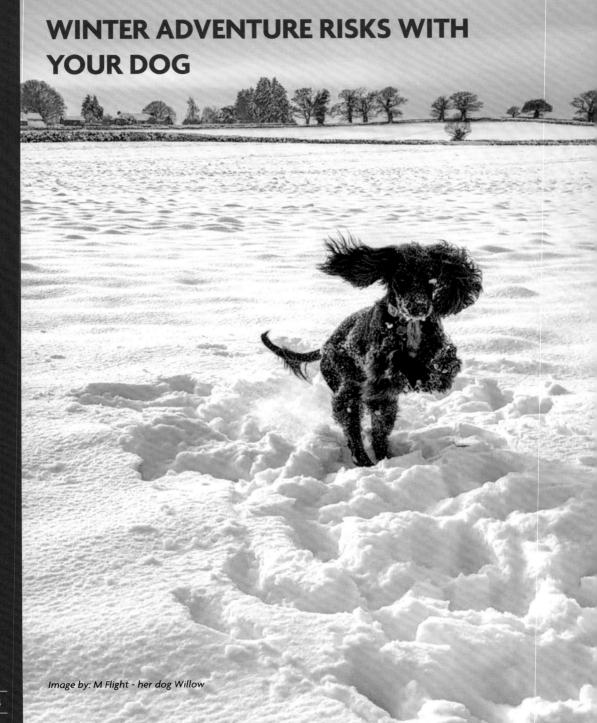

Image by: M Flight - her dog Willow

Hypothermia - When is a dog's temperature too low?

When a dog's body temperature drops to around 98°F or 99°F (37°C), hypothermia is setting in. Hypothermia in dogs — as in humans — is an extreme and dangerous lowering of the body temperature. It happens when pets suffer exposure to freezing temperatures for too long, or if they have wet fur in cold, windy environments. When the body temperature drops, the heart rate and breathing slow down, which can lead to several problems. The consequences of sustained, severe hypothermia may include neurological problems (including coma), heart problems, kidney failure, slow or no breathing, frostbite, and eventually death.

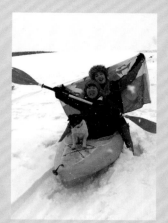

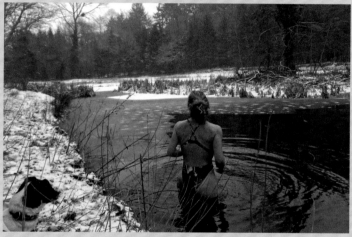

Jack looks on as ice swimming is nice swimming but a definite NO, NO for your woof.

Swimming

Hypothermia during or after swimming can affect dogs as well as humans. The general rule is that if you need to get out of the water because you're getting cold, so does your dog. Ice swimming is totally out of the question with your dog, as they will not recognise a solid surface and will bound onto ice thinking it's safe. I've witnessed far too many situations where a dog has fallen through ice and the distress and panic this brings to dog and owner, let alone the obvious danger to

life. Remember — you are responsible for your pet's health, safety and well-being in ALL conditions and at ALL times.

Frozen Lakes

If you take your dog for walks near a frozen lake take care about letting them off their lead and keep them close to you. Frozen ponds or lakes can be dangerous. Sharp ice could cut their paws, they could slip over and hurt themselves, or they could fall through the ice and drown, or develop hypothermia. Although appearing solid, some frozen lakes may have holes, or areas of thin ice, that your dog could fall into.

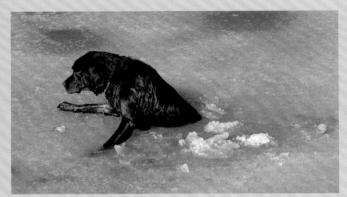

If your dog does fall through ice, do not go in after them. If the ice has broken for your dog then it is likely to break under your weight too. Try to use a long stick, or a leash, to give them something to hold onto, or encourage them to swim to you by calling their name.

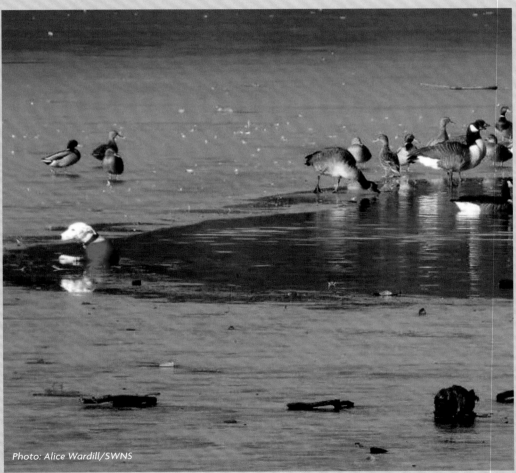

Photo: Alice Wardill/SWNS

Always keep your dog on lead around frozen lakes

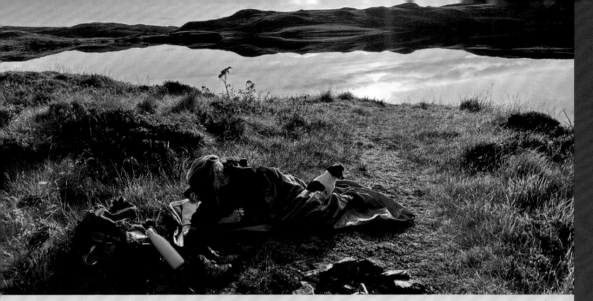

Orkney Islands - Junior and I wake up to Otters having fun.

Winter wild camping – how cold is too cold for a dog to sleep in a tent or Bivvy bag?

Some dogs are simply not built for cold weather camping. Maybe they lack a thick coat as an extra layer of insulation, or maybe they just prefer their creature comforts. Get to know your dog and what they enjoy and what they don't.

For small, old, and short-coated dogs, night-time temperatures below 15.5 degrees are too cold for tent camping without blankets or other protection. For healthy dogs with a thick coat and that are used to colder temperatures, they may even be comfortable camping in temperatures below freezing – if you are!

If you are tough enough to want to wild winter camp, then get your dog used to being out in the cold gradually and invest in a good, warm, waterproof dog coat. Jack used to sleep out in my bivvy bag through summer months and then gradually acclimatise to winter wild camping. He was happy to be my hot water bottle and was the perfect size to snuggle up at my feet in the bivyy bag – but please remember your dog needs good air flow wherever it sleeps.

In an emergency, if you need HELP press your android phone power button 5 times for SOS option.

Please familiarise yourself with these safety options before your adventures.

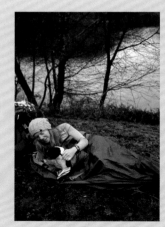

Winter camping is sharing our bivvy bag

Winter is a time to keep your woof out of water.

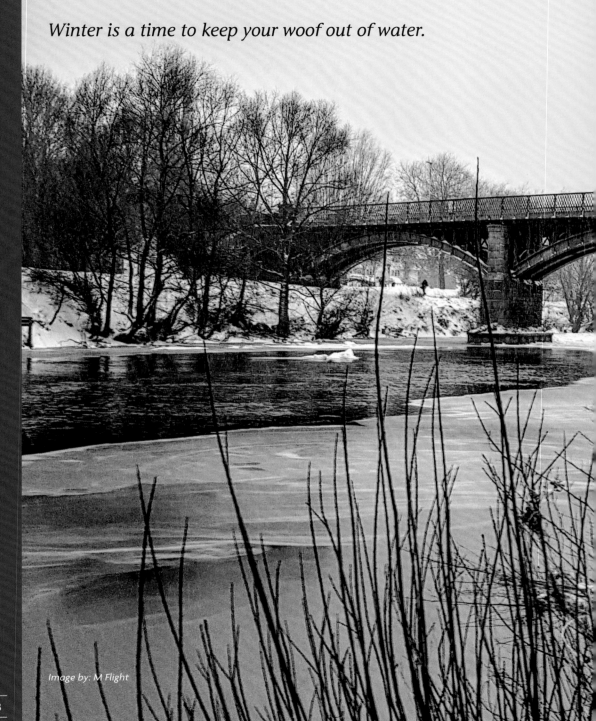

Image by: M Flight

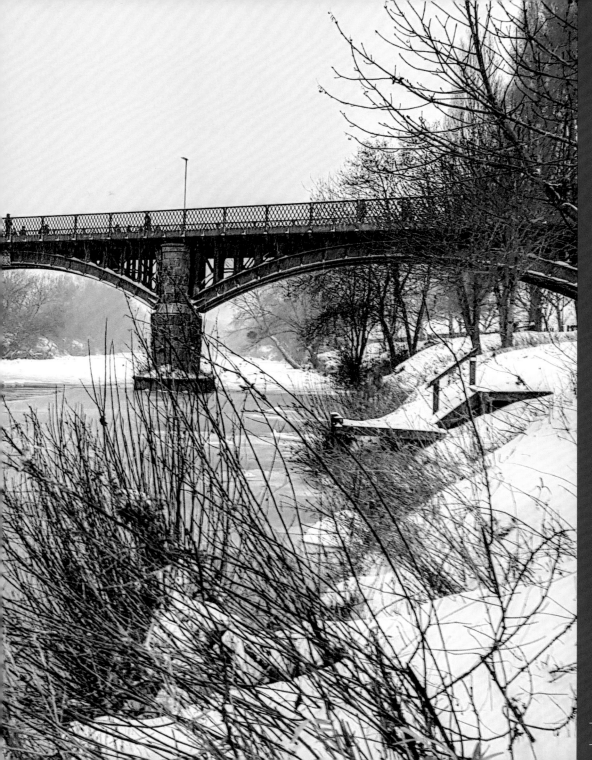

Trails & Mountain walking

Always make sure you have a good understanding of your route and its challenges, like the terrain and possible weather conditions.

Always let someone know where you're going – even if it is a familiar route and you don't plan to be long. Mountain Rescue say that many of their call-outs are to people who know the area well and were just going for a 'short walk'. Make sure you take a good and substantial mountain safety kit for you both.

The age, breed, and health of your dog can all affect the sensitivity to cold weather. Smaller breeds and breeds with a shorter coat are more at risk of frostbite and hypothermia. In cold weather consider investing in a warm coat for your dog. If frosty or there's snow on the ground be extra cautious and only take brief walks. Bigger dogs and breeds with thicker coats can usually withstand lower temperatures. If it's too cold for you it's definitely too cold for your best friend. Just like us, dogs are sensitive to the cold. Dog paws don't freeze because the arrangement of blood vessels beneath the animal's skin keeps the temperature just right, but they can still be uncomfortable and even painful.

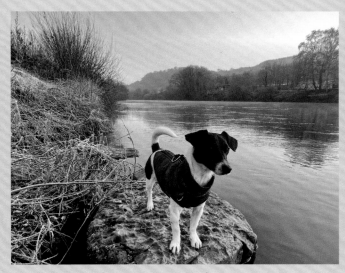

Junior has extra insulation as temperature drops

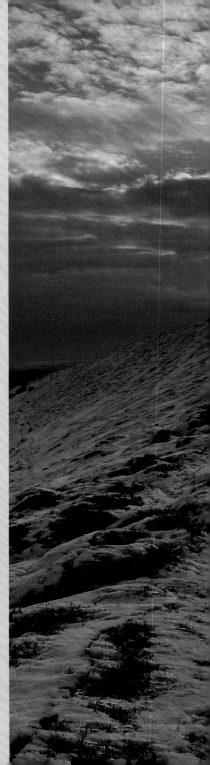

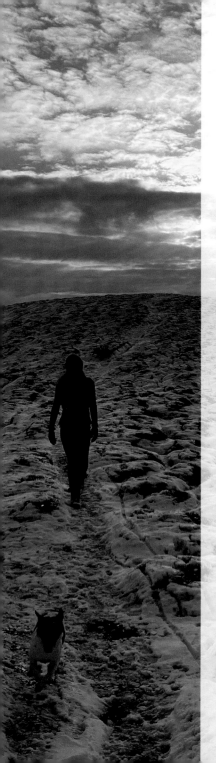

Exposure to cold air, rain and snow can cause chapped paws and dry, itchy skin. Then there are things like ice, chemicals and melting salts that all carry their own dangers and can hurt and harm your dog. There are many substances commonly available in the human world that can prove lethal to your pet. Two to look out for in the winter are antifreeze and rock salt. Both should be kept away from your pet. Always contact your vet immediately if you suspect that your pet has ingested anything that could do them harm.

Winter Kayaking/paddle-boarding

I tend to not take my dog out on the water during the winter months unless it's exceptionally good weather. Cold, wet days when pets risk suffering exposure to freezing temperatures for too long, especially with wet fur in cold, windy environments, is definitely neither safe nor enjoyable for them. Bad weather conditions and short, dark days can provide a cocktail for disaster outdoors.

Winter dangers to dogs

Winter is the season for cold icy weather, dark evening strolls, crunching in the snow and ice, and brisk, frosty walks. These things may be typical signs that winter is with us, but they also indicate a number of seasonal dangers to our dogs. Going out in the cold is all about being prepared, not only in what we wear, but also in knowing what dangers could lie ahead and how to avoid them.

Antifreeze

Antifreeze can be extremely dangerous to dogs. It can damage their kidneys and cause death, even after only a small amount has been licked. It smells and tastes sweet, so may be irresistible to some dogs. Dogs will most often come across it after it's leaked from a car radiator, or been spilt after refilling screen wash. If you notice any liquids by your car, keep your dog away and clean it up immediately. If they've walked through any, then wash their paws with soap and water straight away.

Photo: Black Mountains, Wales

If you think your dog has licked, drunk or been in contact with antifreeze, contact your vet immediately. The quicker your dog is treated the better.

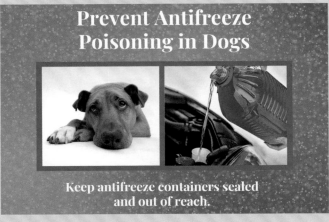

Prevent Antifreeze Poisoning in Dogs

Keep antifreeze containers sealed and out of reach.

paws, stops walking or whines it could be a sign that their paws are too cold. When cold, a dog's body limits blood flow to their extremities (paws, tail, ears etc.) and instead, uses it to keep their vital organs safe and warm. This protects the organs, but does put these extremities at risk of being damaged by the cold. On very cold, icy or snowy days, try to keep the time they spend outside to a minimum and consider using a coat or paw protectors to keep them warm. If you're concerned about them having frostbite contact your vet immediately.

Hypothermia

Very low temperatures and cold winds can quickly reduce your dog's body temperature, causing frostbite and/or hypothermia. Most dogs will be fine outside as they are, but if it's very cold, or if you're spending a bit longer outdoors, then you might want to consider getting a coat for them and some protection for their paws. Every dog is different, but some dogs may be more at risk from cold weather, particularly small, slim, very young or older dogs, or those with short hair. If you do buy a coat make sure it fits well so that it doesn't prevent them moving normally, either through being too tight or too loose. If you're outside in the cold and your pet starts shivering, or appears very tired, then get them home as soon as possible. If they are very unwell, get worse or continue to be unwell, contact your vet immediately.

Frostbite

In very cold weather, if you're out for a walk with your dog, it's important that you keep a close eye on their paws. Ice and snow can stick to the fur between their pads and ball-up. Not only could this be uncomfortable for your dog, but it also increases their risk of frostbite. If your dog lifts their

When a dog's body temperature drops to around 98°F or 99°F (37°C), hypothermia is setting in.

Arthritis

Signs of arthritis can get worse in colder temperatures, so if your dog suffers from this condition they may be stiffer, especially in the morning before they're warmed up.

If you are worried about these signs and if your dog is experiencing any pain, contact your vet.

Winter weight gain

In winter months we are often less active because of the cold wet weather and darker evenings. Getting less exercise means that it's much easier for your dog to put on weight, so it's important to keep an eye on their weight and size.

During the winter you may need to reduce their food portions to prevent them piling on the pounds. Make sure you keep your dog healthy by taking them for regular walks and stay prepared with warmer winter accessories if required.

If you're unable to go out, keep your dog active and entertained by playing indoor games with them.

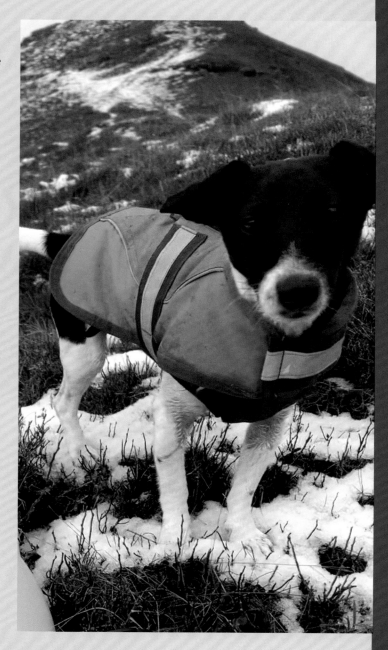

Different breeds have different needs when it comes to winter kit

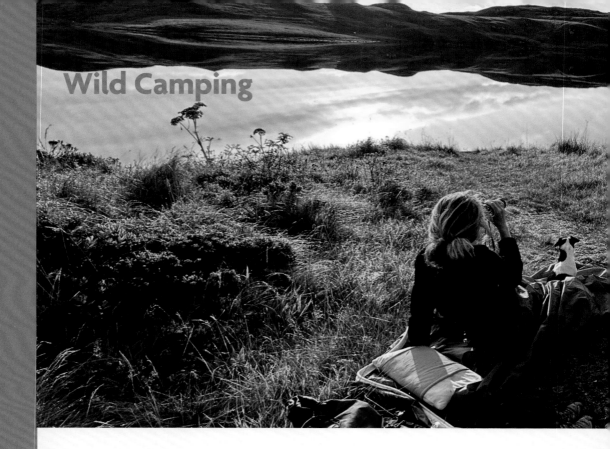

Wild Camping

Wild Camping

Wild Camping has always been part of my life and it's a magical way to connect with Nature.

My dogs have always been part of all my adventures: here Junior enjoys watching a playful early morning otter in the Outer Hebrides, Scotland 2023.

What is wild camping?

'Wild camping' is basically about getting away from the busy commercial campsites and caravan parks, and taking yourself (and your four-legged friend) out into the silent, empty and peaceful wilderness to spend time truly alone with the world.

Sounds fantastic, doesn't it? It is.

There are some specific rules that govern access to wild camping in the UK. The rules are generally split between Scotland and the rest of the country, with Scotland benefiting from open right-to-roam rules. Scotland is indeed the only area of the UK that effectively allows wild camping anywhere, thanks to the Land Reform (Scotland) Act 2003, which permits

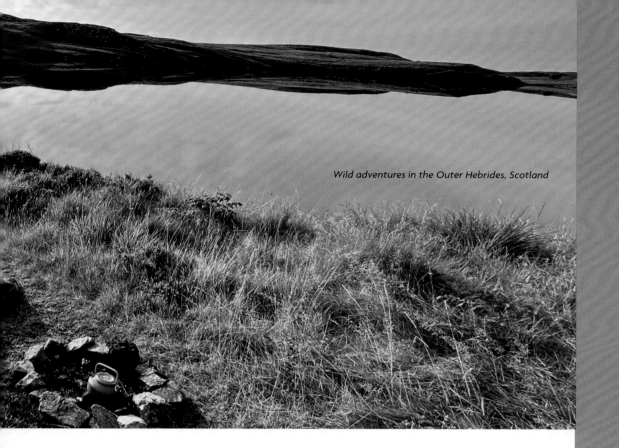

Wild adventures in the Outer Hebrides, Scotland

the public to camp on most unenclosed land. This includes many of Scotland's National Parks, which makes them the perfect destination for wild campers. If you're located in England or Wales, there are still some places where you can go wild camping – such as the Lake District and parts of Dartmoor.

As tempting as it is, you cannot just camp anywhere.

The wild camping UK laws somewhat vary, as it is generally illegal in England and Wales. The general rule for wild camping is that you have to gain permission from the landowner before you pitch up for the night. I always recommend that if you aren't sure you're in a permissible zone, you should check first, as you could be disturbing farmland or private property.

All land is owned by someone so if you are 'allowed' to use it, be sure to be courteous and respectful. In other words, keep your groups small, keep your fires small, and take your rubbish home with you. It's good manners to be polite and respectful of other people's land and most farmers and landowners will thank you for it.

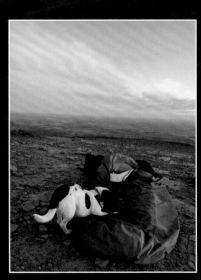

Jack gets ready to bed down for the night
on Penyfan where we watch the sun set
and rise for the summer solstice.

"Our imagination for the wild FEEDS our adventurous lives"

A. Jones

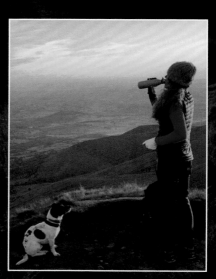

Hiking in the Brecon Beacons our homeland is a particular favourite of ours.

Guidelines for wild camping

If you have decided that wild camping is for you, it is important to follow some basic rules to ensure that you leave as little trace behind as possible. 'Take only memories and leave only foot-prints'. After all, Nature is exactly that – natural. Your wild camping trip should leave no impact on the landscape and shouldn't disturb the environment or wildlife around you. Here are a few rules and wild camping tips and tricks to remember:

1. Follow the Scottish Outdoor Access Code if you are wild camping in Scotland. This code covers three basic principles for sharing the countryside with others: respecting the interests of other people, caring for the environment, and taking responsibility for your own actions.

2. Leave no trace of your stay. This is especially important if you are wild camping in national parks and on protected landscapes, as the area should be kept pristine for everyone to enjoy. Don't leave any rubbish behind, always clear up any mess you have made and ensure that you don't disturb wildlife.

3. Don't light any fires, even if there are signs that fires have previously been lit in the same area. Lighting fires can not only be dangerous but will also spoil the landscape and leave a trace of your visit. Use camping stoves and portable barbecues carefully, ensuring that you don't scorch any grass.

4. Be respectful with your 'personal' waste. If you are camping out in the wilderness, you will inevitably need to go to the toilet. But that doesn't mean that you can just go anywhere! Make sure that you go to the toilet well away from any natural streams or rivers and bury anything you might leave behind with a shovel or trowel. Feminine hygiene products should be treated like rubbish and taken away with you – animals can dig them up if buried, which won't be pleasant for people to come across later and can even be hazardous to wildlife.

5. Don't be an eyesore or a nightmare! When other people are out walking and hiking, they want to enjoy the landscape as much as you do. You should, therefore, make sure that you don't take over the view with a large tent or 'camp'. Be considerate and blend in with your surroundings as much as possible.

6. HAVE FUN!
Taking your dog camping for the first time is exciting, but it might feel a little daunting too. Do your best to prepare ahead of time and have a back-up plan to mitigate some of those nerves. But, beyond that, a little patience and sense of humour will always help. Not all dogs take to sleeping in a tent (or going in and out of tent doors) right away, but with practice and patience they will get the hang of it.

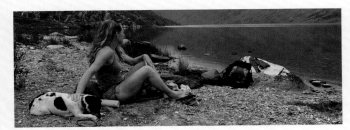

Glenbeg Lough, Ireland

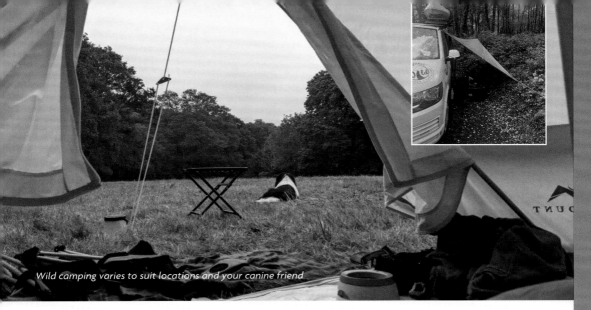

Wild camping varies to suit locations and your canine friend

Remember that part of what makes camping such fun is that things rarely go exactly as planned. That's just part of the adventure and these things always make great stories afterwards. As long as everyone is safe, you're making memories together and building your bonds – whether human or canine – and that's undeniably fun!

So, relax, don't stress and keep giving plenty of happy vibes to your dog. Introducing your dog to your camping kit before your adventure will help them become comfortable with these 'new things'. Get them used to seeing you with a rucksack and unfolding your sleeping kit, try setting it out in the garden or for a picnic in the woods – but not sleeping out at first. Show them how you snuggle up in your tent and bivvy bag – you can cwtch up in the bivvy bag in your own front room! Teach them how much fun it is to chill out and just relax together. Obviously the size of the dog will dictate if they can join you in the bivvy bag and/or tent. As I have mentioned, my little Jack would sleep between the sleeping bag and bivvy bag down by my feet. Always make sure your dog has enough airflow if they are going to jump into a bivvy bag. I always used to take Jack's blanket – the one that he associated with wild camping – so he had the 'head's up' that we were going on an adventure. We were both normally pretty tired at the end of a day, so he was happy to curl up and have those special cuddles that he wouldn't normally give at home. It was a true bond of trust and our special place where we felt at one and as one.

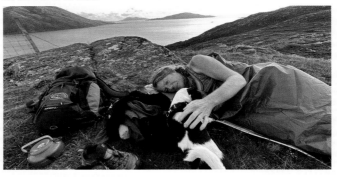

Wild Scottish Isles

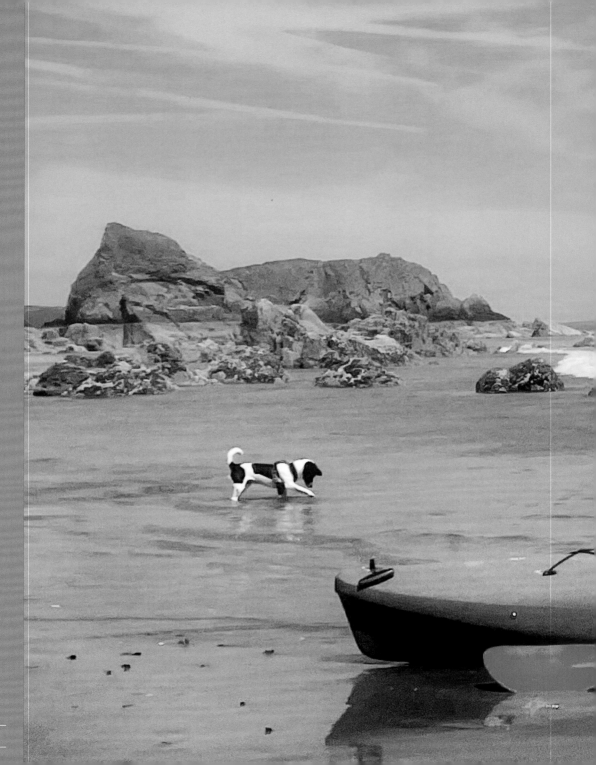

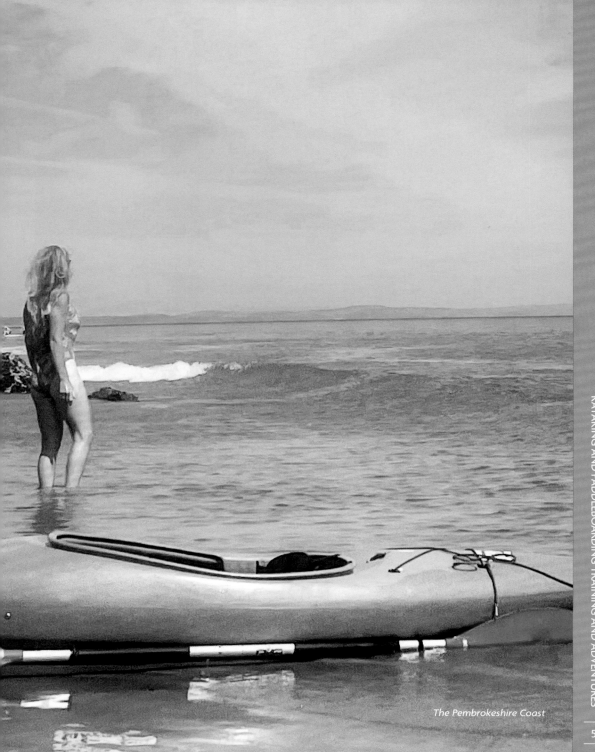

The Pembrokeshire Coast

Kayaking and paddle-boarding with your dog

You might love and be experienced in Outdoor paddling adventures but first, you need to think about safety and whether your dog is ready and able to join you on the water. They should be a comfortable, confident swimmer. Some dogs take to water instantly and were even bred for it, such as Newfoundlands and Labrador Retrievers. These are going to be much easier to train. Others aren't so happy and confident and need a lot more extra help to get them settled on your boat or board.

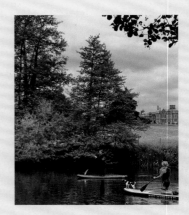

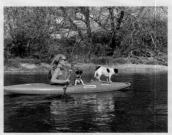

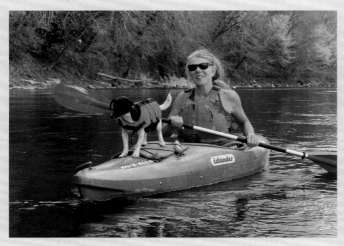

Similarly, if your dog is very energetic, playful, and has trouble listening in new environments, you might need to devote more training time before heading out on the water. Or perhaps your dog is quite timid and nervous. If so, think about if kayaking, canoeing or paddleboarding is for them. It is about what suits your dog, not what suits you.

We know, hopefully, that we are not silly enough to be hurtling down rapids and manoeuvring around jagged rocks, but even the gentle bobbing of the boat and splashing of the paddles might distress very anxious dogs, and make them feel out of control. Know your dog and their boundaries.

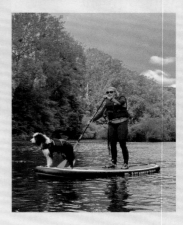

Know your dog and their limits

BEFORE YOU START

Similar to kayaking and canoeing, paddle boarding can be an overwhelming experience for your dog. Things as simple as wearing a life jacket or standing on the board can increase fear if these experiences are new and unnatural to them. To make the transition as smooth as possible, use these tips to introduce your dog to the sport before getting on the water.

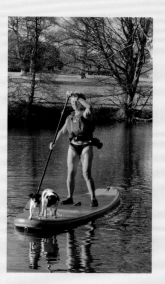

1. Teach your dog basic cues (page 56)
Before you and your dog get out on the water, make sure they have mastered basic obedience cues like "sit" and "stay". This will make you and your dog more confident and therefore safer.

2. Master your paddle board
Don't get on a SUP with your dog until you're confident using one by yourself. You should be comfortable standing up, paddling, and turning. Make sure you can also fall in the water and get back on easily. Dogs will mirror your stress if you are not comfortable, and being on a stand up paddle board with a dog in tow will only make things more difficult and stressful for beginners.

3. Introduce your dog and board (page 56)
Before hitting the water, introduce your dog to the board on solid ground – just like the kayak or canoe. Put the board in an area of the house, or outside, where your dog is comfortable. Allow them to sniff it, look at it, and explore it on their own terms. It's not a problem if they don't jump right on at first – it's just there for them to get used to. Use treats on and around the board to encourage them to explore it and to make it fun.

4. Teach the behaviour you want on the board (page 57)
You can train this by teaching the dog to stay on a mat and move it onto the board, or you can work directly on the board. Encourage your dog to walk on using treats, ask them to sit or lie down and give more treats.

5. Practice cues for getting off the board
Before you get out on the water, practice a special cue for getting off the board, and only reward your dog when they jump off on cue. If they get off without the cue, lead them back on the board and try again. After a while, they should get the hang of it. A lot of the time dogs get excited and jump off the board when you're getting close to shore. This can throw you off balance and into the water, which can be more dangerous near the shore.

6. Do a dry run
When they're comfortable, put on their life jacket and get them on the board again. If you do this several times, standing on the board with their life jacket will feel more natural. The only difference when you are out on the water will be the surroundings.

7. Make sure your dog is fit and can swim

Before paddleboarding with your dog, ensure they are comfortable strong swimmers. You may not intend for them to end up in the water but all might not go to plan and you must be prepared. If they are a weak swimmer or afraid of water, the experience will not be enjoyable and could even be dangerous. As a pet parent your dog's safety is your responsibility.

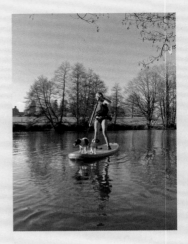

8. Trim sharp nails

Anyone who has ever swum near a dog knows that shorter nails are better than long, sharp ones. By keeping your dog's nails short and dull, you will minimise the chance of the finish of your board getting scratched, or your deck pad torn.

9. Bring a pocket full of treats

Bring treats out on your adventure so you can continue to reward good behaviour and maintain training.

10. Tire out energetic pups

Balancing on a SUP is very tiring for dogs, but a very energetic dog will be unlikely to keep still. Play a short game of fetch or go for a short walk or swim together before getting on the board to both warm up their muscles and take a little excess zip out of your dog. This will make them a better more relaxed passenger and less likely to throw both of you into the water.

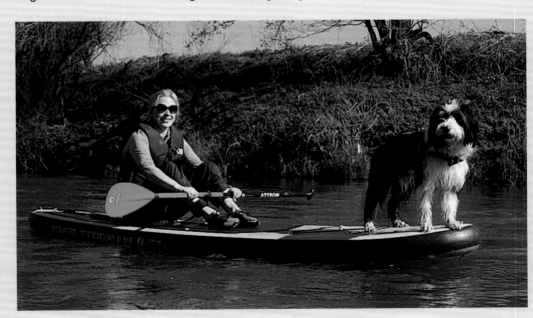

Best Paddle-boards for dogs

The best paddle boards for dogs are the wider and longer boards because they are more stable in the water. When you're choosing a paddle board for you and your dog, it's best to look at a board that is at least ten feet long and 32 inches wide. Boards over ten feet long are the most stable, which makes them a good choice when you're taking your dog along for the ride.

When choosing a board, make sure you consider your weight, as well as the weight of your dog. The larger the dog in comparison to the board, the more unstable it will be. Paddle boarding with large dogs is not a problem as long as you have the right board. Part of making sure your board is woof-ready is to select a board with a full deck pad for safe traction.

Many paddle boards don't provide much grip for your dog's paws. Get a paddle board with dog-friendly grip to make sure your buddy doesn't go sliding off when you hit a wave. The best SUPs (stand up paddle boards) for dogs are boards that have a full deck pad, or at least an extended deck pad. Inflatable boards typically come with extended deck pads. If your board does not have a large enough deck pad, there are other options. Old yoga mats or bath mats with suction cups are great alternatives. And remember dogs' paws are very sensitive and can easily overheat and burn on hot surfaces like SUPs and kayaks.

Most dogs are naturally good swimmers, but since the paddle board adds an element that your pooch isn't familiar with, it's a good idea to get them a life jacket. A dog jumping off a tipping paddle board could easily get disoriented and get swept away. Put the life jacket on your dog at home first to make sure it fits properly and so they can get used to it before going in the water.

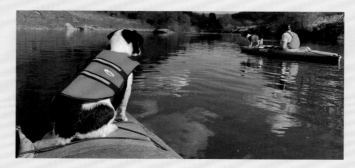

Best Kayaks for Dogs

Rather than an enclosed cockpit a sit on top kayak is ideal for dogs as it has a broad area for seating, which makes it easier if you and your dog need to capsize. If you have larger dogs consider a tandem kayak. Personally, I've always used leisure kayaks that are very stable with a large cockpit for that all-important kit, and they have a large bow (front of kayak) and stern (back of kayak) as my woofs have always been small dogs and balance extremely well on the bow. I always add a non-slip padded mat on the bow section for my woof for comfort and safety and protecting those paws.

I would never recommend that dogs ever go into the cockpit just in case you capsize and they get caught underneath. Never tie your dog up by a leash on your raft. I've seen this so many times and it absolutely haunts me. There has been a worrying increase in dogs drowning as water adventures with your dog increases.

How to prepare your dog

Introducing the equipment

If you think your dog will enjoy joining you on the water, a major step along the road to kayaking, canoeing or paddleboarding with them safely is getting them accustomed to your boat or board. You can try this by putting it in the house or garden and letting them sniff around it before putting them inside or on it.

If they seem nervous or wary of the boat, take your time and watch them. When they move towards it, put one of their favourite treats close to it. Watch and wait for them to get a little bit closer in their own relaxed time. Spend a few minutes doing this and then have a break and try again later. You really don't need to get them on the boat the first time, but reducing the pressure on them and giving them choice is the quickest way to build their confidence and make progress. Keep your sessions short and positive and you'll have a confident boat dog in no time.

Many dogs are sensitive to loud noises, and inflatable paddle boards can be extremely noisy. If you can expose them to this noise gradually it will help. For the first time try it at a distance where you are confident that it will not worry them and make sure it happens while they are busy engaging in a different fun activity. If they seem happy with this then the next time you can bring them a little closer. It's better to start off cautiously

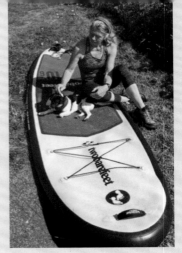

Junior gets familiarised with board

than risk scaring your dog and putting them off.

If they don't seem interested, try getting in the boat or on the board too and let them follow you, or scatter some of their favourite toys or treats in and around it to encourage them. It's all about trust and familiarity. They need to know it's safe – for you as well as them!

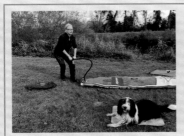
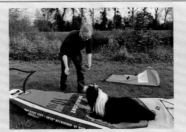
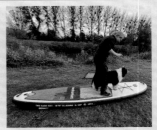

Get your dog used to the paddleboard gently as the sound of inflating and deflating can be quite noisy and stressful. Pixel learns to wait on the training mat, then gently moves on to the board and learns the paddling position with an important treat as a reward.

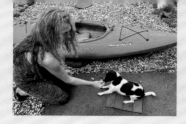
Junior gets used to his kayak mat in the garden

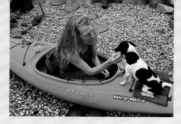
Place mat on kayak; add treats

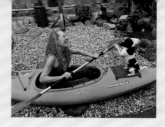
Fun time getting used to equipment

Once they get their scent on it, and see it as a fun thing to do, it'll make it a lot easier for your dog to feel comfortable when it comes to heading out on the water. Making sure you have your pet's favourite treats handy and that you reward them every time they listen will definitely help.

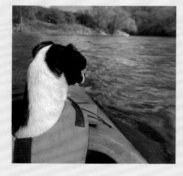

Training behaviours

Cue Training is crucial when it comes to kayaking, canoeing or paddleboarding with dogs. When you're out on the water, it's critical that your dog does exactly what you tell it to, should you run into difficulty. This is where your earlier land training will come in. There will also probably be a lot of wildlife nearby, so there's a good chance that your dog will want to leap overboard from sheer excitement. My dogs never get to go out on water till they've learnt to respect wildlife.

They should already know 'stay' and 'come back', teach them and proof these behaviours so that they can still listen in distracting and difficult environments. Learning these two key cues means they'll remain on your boat – regardless of distractions – and also that they'll return when you let them go off for a swim or run about the shore during an all important break. Even if your dog may already know these cues, they could react differently on the water, which is why proofing in different places alongside different distractions is key. Before you go kayaking, paddleboarding or canoeing with a dog, take them to your planned paddling area and try out your cues by the water's edge. This will help your dog make a connection between these cues and the paddling environment and help them get used to the movement of the water.

To help your dog to learn that you want it to stay on the boat or board while paddling, you can start by training it to stay on a mat. To begin this, you need a new mat that the dog has no previous experience with. Give the dog treats for staying on the mat and teach a cue for getting off the mat by only rewarding the dog for getting off after you have asked them to. When your dog understands that when the mat is out they get treats for staying on it, you can begin to proof this by increasing the distractions around them and by taking it to new environments. You can then put the mat on the boat or board to help your dog to learn that you want the same behaviour there.

Whilst it can be great fun being on the water with your four-legged friend, there are a few points to keep in mind before you head out onto the water.

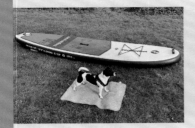
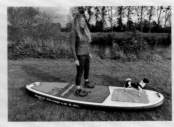

Body confidence, core strength and balance

Balancing on a kayak or SUP while it bobs in the water takes a lot of strength and balance, even in gentle conditions and even if you stand on four paws. The dog needs to be happy moving on different surfaces, including slippery ones, and have good "proprioception" (i.e. the dog knowing where its limbs are in space). Dogs are typically very good at knowing where their front end is, but they don't pay too much attention to their back end as they can't see it as well as the front and it just seems to follow along. In everyday life this is completely fine, but on a kayak or SUP it could cause them to misplace their back paw and fall off.

The good news is that paddling with your pup should help with all of these things, and developing these skills will help your dog stay healthy, fit, and confident in other areas of their life.

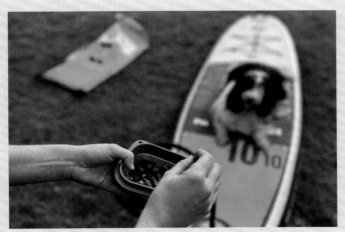

One approach would be to introduce your dog to paddling slowly, with lots of short but frequent sessions, gradually building in duration when you are sure that the dog is happy and strong. However, you might not have access to your own kayak or SUPs all of the time; you may have an inflatable that is packed away, or you may not want to go paddling all year round! Luckily, we can practice these skills without any special equipment, with things you can find on walks or with furniture and other household items. If you're feeling particularly keen then you can buy or make special fitness equipment, but all you really need is a dog and a bag of tasty treats.

When doing fitness training we are aiming for movement to be slow, controlled, and precise. It's better to have a few good quality movements than to overdo it. The last thing you want is for your dog to be sore and uncomfortable and not want to do any more training. There are lots of exercises that you can do to help with core strength and balance, just like for humans, but here are a few to get you started:

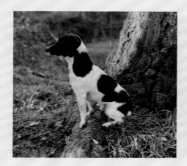 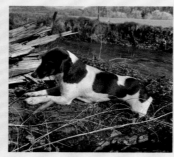 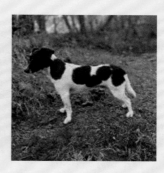

1. Doggy push ups

Exactly as with human push ups, it takes more strength to do it slowly than quickly. Even if your dog knows how to do a 'sit', 'down', or possibly even a 'stand', when doing fitness training you can slow them down by luring them with treats, exactly like when you first taught them. It's important to check for good posture – the positions should be straight and not leaning to one side or the other. It can help to use a platform that is only a little bigger than the dog, to give them a clear physical indicator to stay straight by staying on the platform. Don't do too many repetitions of these as they're hard work!

- Ask for a 'sit' and lift the treat upwards from their nose.
- Ask for a 'down' and bring the treat diagonally forwards and down.
- Ask for a 'sit' and lift the treat upwards.

You can also do this with a 'down' to 'stand':

- From a standing position, ask for a 'down' and with the treat on their nose, move it diagonally down and backwards (into them).

You're looking for them to fold back like a sphinx.

- From the 'down', ask for a 'stand' and with the treat on their nose, move it diagonally forwards and upwards. You're aiming for them to keep all four paws still while their body lifts upwards into position.

Standing straight

With the dog in a well-balanced, straight stand position you can lift a paw one at a time. Remember to give lots of treats, balancing on three legs is hard work. You can also gently push the side of the dog and give them treats for staying in position and pushing back against you. Some dogs may

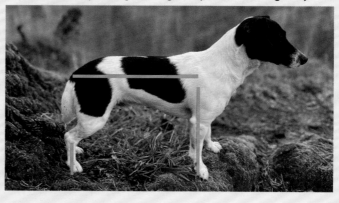

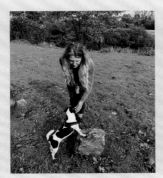
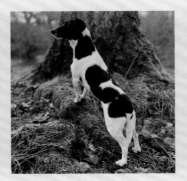
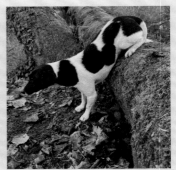

think you want them to move when you gently push them; if that happens then you need to go back to feeding them for standing without being pushed and slowly introduce the other hand.

2. Paws up & pivots

Getting your dog to put their paws up onto objects can help to increase their body confidence, especially if you use a variety of different items and surfaces in lots of different places. You can use big logs, rocks, park benches, anything! Make sure that they are stable and safe before asking your dog to put their weight on. You can use treats as a lure to start with and then put it on a cue.

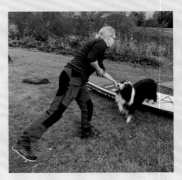

3. Where are my back feet?

This one is great for strength and proprioception. You need to find a large-ish stable object (like a SUP! Or a platform) and ask your dog to

When your dog is happy putting their paws onto objects you may want to get them pivoting around the object – that's keeping their front paws on while moving their back paws around. For this you want an object that is very stable, non-slip, and not too high off the ground. This is great for strengthening core muscles and hips. Start by feeding the dog for being in front of you with his paws on the object, then take a small step left or right around the object. Your dog will probably naturally want to stand in front of you and will reposition itself to do so. To start with, reward the dog for any back leg movement that mirrors yours (even if it's teeny tiny!) and as its confidence builds so will the speed and precision.

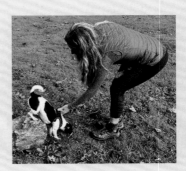

walk over it. When its front paws are off but its back paws are still on, mark and reward. Give it a few extra treats for staying in that position and then use a release cue (or the one you want to use for getting off the board) and throw a treat away to reset. Repeat this until your dog knows that it gets treats for putting its back paws on the object and then you can put a verbal cue on it. You can even turn it into walking backwards by positioning the dog with the object just behind it and giving your verbal cue.

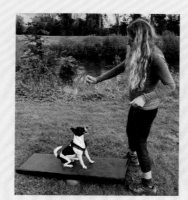
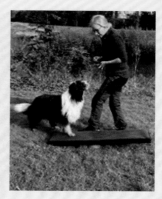

4.Obstacle course

Kayaks and SUPs are wobbly in the water and your dog might not have walked on unstable surfaces before. We can make this fun and practice at home in all weather by creating obstacle courses for our dogs. See what you can find that they can safely walk on, try lots of different materials and surfaces, and when they're confident with this you can introduce a wobble by putting cushions under hard (non-slip) surfaces. Be as creative as you like!

Remember that doing this slowly in a controlled way is key, so once you've set up your obstacle course, use treats to lure your dog over, making sure that they put their feet on each object in turn rather than jumping over and slipping off. You might discover that your dog doesn't like certain textures – in which case don't push it, it's meant to be fun. Build their confidence on surfaces that they like and then introduce new ones slowly. You can also try this outside using park benches and other natural features.

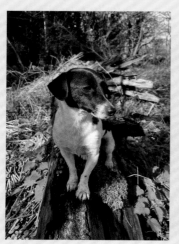
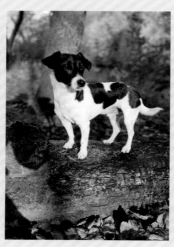
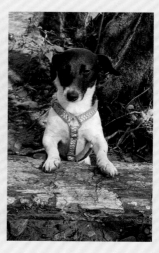

FITNESS TIPS

1. Confidence is king

Some dogs are happy to fling themselves around without a care in the world and others might be more hesitant to put their paws on new objects. If your dog is more hesitant then you might have to start slowly and let them get used to a specific new object that you want them to put their paws on. When they think this is really fun you can start to move the behaviour to other surfaces. Never force your dog to do something they aren't comfortable with; confidence builds by letting them make choices and celebrating them, not by forcing discomfort.

2. Quality not quantity

Getting a few very good reps is much better than getting lots of sloppy ones. Going for high reps could risk injuring your dog, taking the fun out of the exercise, and not working the right muscle groups.

3. Slow and steady

Doing exercises slowly is much harder than doing them quickly. Try luring your dog to slow down if they're going too fast.

4. Little and often

Doing a few exercises regularly will get you a much better result than long sessions every once in a while; will keep it fun, and will reduce the risk of pushing your dog too hard.

5. Tiny tasty treats

When you do exercises like these you can go through a lot of treats. If you make them small then your dog can have lots and lots without feeling too full to keep going.

6. Check for signs of injury and overdoing it

Always pay attention when your dog is exercising; check for repeated irregular movement and stop if you see something that you don't like. Likewise, if your dog is doing a lot more stretching than normal afterwards, you probably overdid it. Give them rest and try to keep the sessions shorter in future.

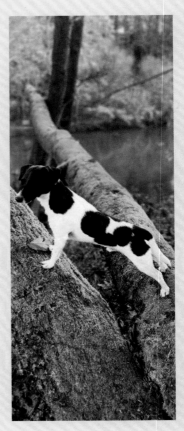

If your dog doesn't want to do the exercises, listen and stop. They could be sore, injured, or nervous.

Try again another day and if an issue persists you may need to visit a Vet Physio.

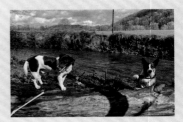

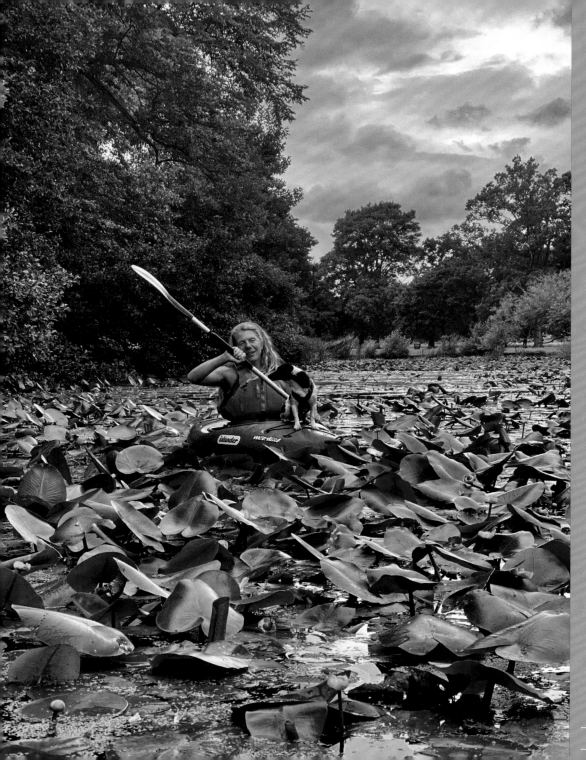

HOW TO PADDLE BOARD WITH YOUR DOG

1. Warm up your dog. Balancing on a board is hard work for them; take them for a 5-minute walk or play to warm up those muscles before you start.

2. Have your dog stay on shore as you go out on the board on your own. Wave to it, laugh, and smile so they know that it is fun and not scary.

3. Hold the board still in shallow water and allow your dog to get on. Walk the board through the shallow water and allow them to jump off if they want.

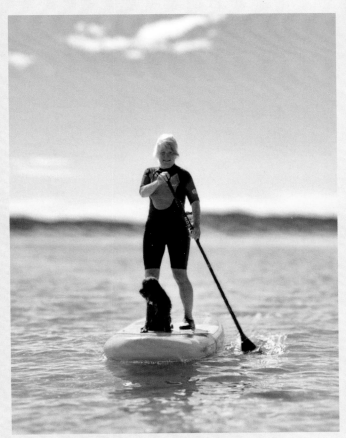

Jill starts out in shallow, calm waters intrducing her dog gently.

4. When you're both ready, get onto the board with your dog. Start out paddling on your knees for better balance.

5. Stand up with your dog between or at your feet. Get used to paddling without accidentally hitting them with the paddle.

6. Small dogs can sit on the nose of the board. Once you've mastered keeping the paddle away from your dog, they can sit in front of you on the board. For better weight distribution and balance, large dogs can sit on the back third of the board.

Make sure that you balance the board, so if the dog is at the front, you will need to stand a little behind the centre, and if the dog is at the back you should be standing a little towards the front of centre.

7. Keep it short the first time out. When you get back to shore, reward your dog and give it praise. It may not go perfectly the first time out, but it's all part of the learning experience.

8. Be prepared for your dog to jump off at any time. The board will move a lot when a large dog jumps off, and when it happens you may fall in as well. Make sure that you're only standing on the board

when in deep enough water and away from any hazards like boats or people.

9. If your dog jumps or falls off the board, help them back on. This will help make sure they don't scratch the board's finish trying to get on. Life jackets will usually have handles for you to help them aboard.

10. Take drinking water out for both of you. If you are paddling on the ocean, your dog might try to drink the salt water. Taking in too much salt water can cause further dehydration (and other health issues).

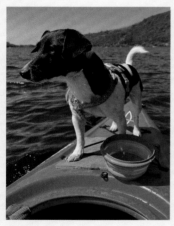

BIGGEST TIP, BE PATIENT Not all dogs were born to ride. If it isn't clicking, don't force it. Getting frustrated will make the experience unpleasant for both of you.

SAFETY TIPS FOR PADDLING

• Take a First Aid kit – and know how to use it. Never go out for hours on end. Always, have a small First Aid kit. Paddle boarding should be fun and relaxing – you don't want to be rushing back to treat minor injuries. First Aid kits can also help you make temporary repairs to torn or damaged equipment.

• Apply sunscreen to your dog (and yourself). Please apply environmentally friendly cream that does NOT harm aquatic life and remember our sunscreen is toxic for dogs. Dogs are at risk of sunburn just like humans, especially on their bellies. Some dogs have a very thin layer of fur in that area and can be burned by sunlight reflected off the water. Apply sunscreen to any exposed areas and do not spend more than a couple of hours in the sun at a time.

• Kneel or sit near hazards. Only stand on the board when in open water and away from rocks, boats, people, and any other potential hazards. This is always recommended when paddleboarding alone, and not just when you're with your dog. However, it is especially applicable with a pooch that could throw you off your balance at any time.

• Add a life jacket and always unclip their lead. If you fall into the water their lead could get caught on rocks or even around the board. It's much safer for them if they can be trained to stay on the board without a lead, so they either swim back to you or paddle to dry land should they fall in.

• Rinse your dog after your adventure. Paws and skin can be irritated by salt. After being in the water always rinse your dog off, and make sure not to neglect the ears (without getting water in the ears). Ear infections can result if water is left trapped in your dog's ears.

• Be aware of hazards If you are at the sea: sea-lice can irritate dogs and jellyfish can pose a hazard for both of you. Hot sand can also harm your dog's paws. If it is standing on the beach, try to keep your pup in the shade or even in ankle-deep water.

• Never leave your dog in a vehicle. All dog owners should know this, but it's always worth repeating. In warm weather, it can only take a matter of minutes for a dog to get heat stroke if left in a car unattended. Only have pets in the car if you're in there with them, with the windows open or air conditioning on.

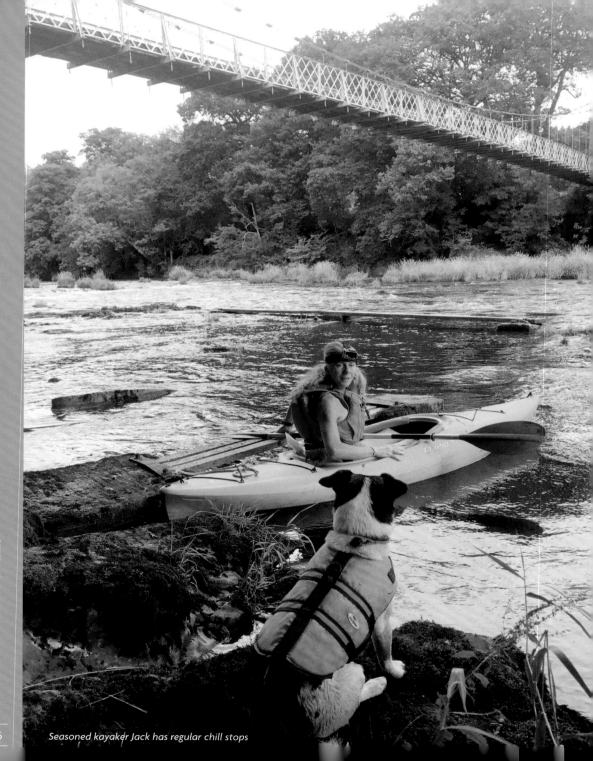

Seasoned kayaker Jack has regular chill stops

LAUNCHING YOUR BOAT

Get your dog to sit in (or on) the boat (or board) as you push it away from shore. Repeating this until you're seated in the boat yourself is a good way to keep dogs calm, and it should help persuade them to remain on board and not run to you in a panic.

Once you're both on board and away from the shore, gently start moving the oars to propel you both forwards – but be very gentle. Dogs scare easily in new surroundings, and accidentally banging the side of the boat or splashing your pet might just cause them to panic. After a slow and steady paddling motion, your dog should relax, and then you can confidently say you're canoeing, paddleboarding or kayaking with your dog!

Always start with a short shallow paddle close to shore, then gradually increase your distance.

ALWAYS PUT YOUR DOG FIRST AS YOUR LIMIT MAY BE PAST YOUR DOG'S.

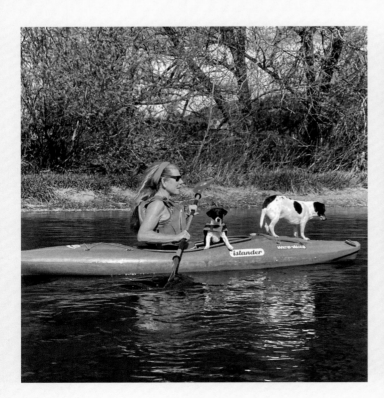

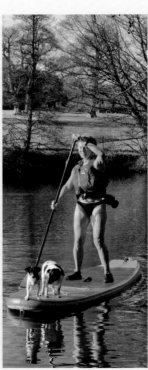

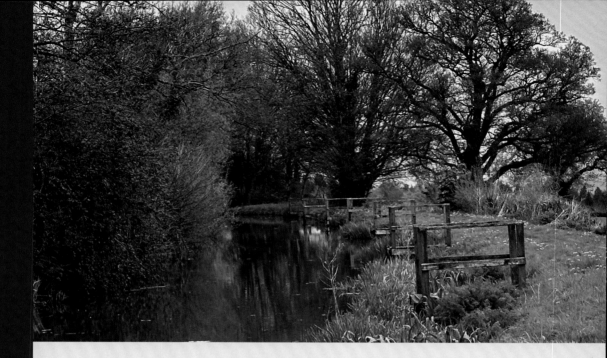

Dogs and biking

How to get started safely

Trails are safer and more pleasurable than the roads for both two legs and four, and it is also gentler on the dog's skeletal system as they run alongside.

I've always enjoyed biking with my dogs. All my dogs have been Jack Russell terriers, so they're easy to put into a pet carrier when you feel they need a rest, which allows you to go on longer rides and cover more miles. The carry case also stores that all important doggy kit, snacks, a lead, water and a rain cover.

Please remember that a dog is still growing and developing physically for the first 18 months of its life so it is important not to over exercise and stress the joints.

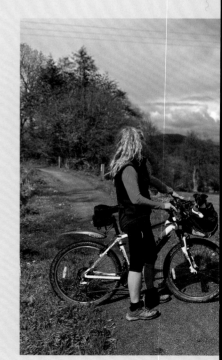

Biking the Brecon Canal, trails are so much safer and pleasurable.

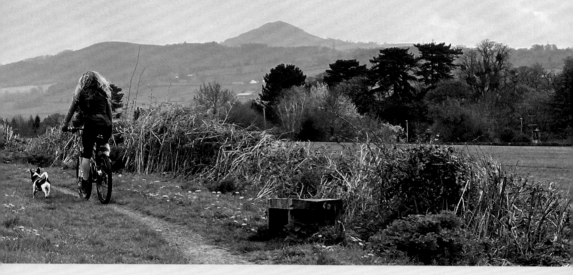

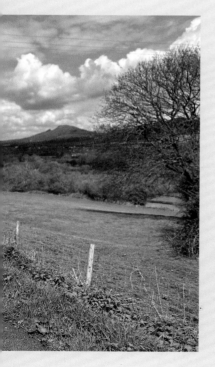

1. Start by getting them to go for walks where you will see other bikers on trail paths. This will enable you to teach them 'bike manners' – avoiding the path of the other cyclists and not to chase them.
2. For the next stage I always push my bike while walking with my dog to teach them to walk by my side and so they can get familiar and comfortable with this strange lump of metal on wheels, the pet carrier and bell.
3. Then I take a short 5-minute ride with the dog running alongside. This can gradually be built up to suit your best friend.

It is essential that you pace your bike ride to suit your dog's fitness level (not yours), its size and breed.

Small-to-medium dogs cannot keep up with fast moving bikes nor endure long distances because of their shorter legs and bio-mechanics, so always adapt your ride to suit your best friend's needs and enjoyment.

99% of my bike journeys are on trails. I very rarely bike on road and if I do I always put my dog in the pet carrier. Your dog's safety is paramount at all times.

It's best to only take healthy, large dogs to run alongside you for longer bike rides.

Biking is not like playing in the garden for hours, it takes lots of energy, is a big adventure and therefore should be built up slowly. Try 5-10 minutes in the first week for rides and runs, and gradually increase from there.

Running on hard surfaces can be damaging to a dog's physical health, so dogs must be properly conditioned before heading out for longer rides. Always monitor how your dog copes and adjust the outing accordingly.

There is no law to say that you and your dog are not allowed to ride on the road, but section 68 of The Highway Code says it is illegal to ride a bike in a "dangerous, careless or inconsiderate manner." Of course, there is no reason to ever do that anyway.

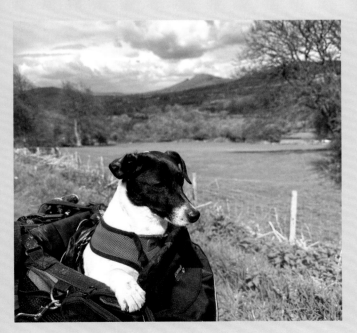

Carrying your dog on your bike

- The front basket – best for getting out the door quickly and shorter sessions.
- The bike cargo trailer – best for bigger breeds or multiple dogs.
- The rear basket– best for longer journeys.
- The bike leash – best for adventures

Getting your dog used to a pet carrier

Get them used to seeing the pet carrier around the home first so it loses any fear for them. Then get them to go in and out, familiarising themselves with the item and building up a trust, knowing it is a safe space.

Gradually, build up to attaching the pet carrier to thebike so your dog knows it is going on the trips with you! It is all about getting your dog used to different things and it's best to do this in gradual stages to gain trust. A good trick to get your dog used to the bike is to praise your dog and make them feel included and happy whenever the bike is around.

How to cycle with your dog by your side

Always match the pace of your dog, rather than the other way around. Let them set the pace. Be mindful of the temperature and when it changes. Don't over exert your dog. Make sure your bike brakes are in good condition in case you need to do an emergency stop – even the best behaved dog can make mistakes! For this reason, make sure you keep your dog behind or to the side of the bike – never in front.

I recommend that once your dog is fit enough to run a distance of around 2 miles comfortably, you should limit biking to every other day to provide a day of rest for rejuvenation of the muscles. Extremely fit dogs can run greater distances each day if the sessions are broken up. Always reduce the distance if riding on a pavement, which like the road, can be tough on the skeletal system.

Remember that dogs are predators – even your cuddly little pet; they may naturally want to chase prey. This is where your earlier training to accept and respect wildlife and not to chase it will pay off.

Anything that moves faster than the dog will appear to be prey as the dog interprets it as 'flight' or 'fleeing'. Therefore, instinct will often kick in and the chase is on!

That innate 'prey drive' can be irresistible to the dog, so it is important to have certain skills, like ignoring prey, ingrained in your dog from an early age.

It is even more important to perfect before you cycle, so that any wildlife you may meet won't send your dog into a frenzy and tip you off the bike.

Unfortunately, you may meet other aggressive dogs on your bike rides. If you can't deter the dog and you feel that confrontation is inevitable then stop, put the bike between you and the aggressive dog and avoid eye contact.

Having an 'air horn' or 'repellent' can really make a difference as it deflects the aggressive dog's attention.

Bike leashes are better for bigger dog adventures.

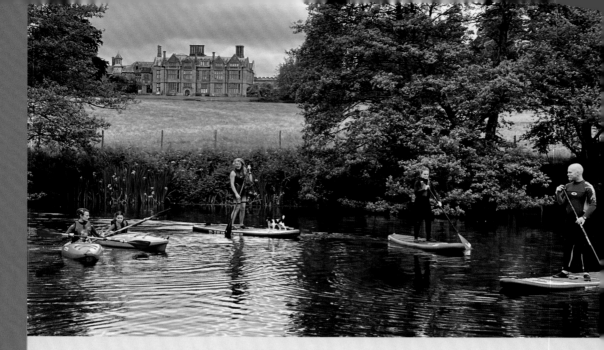

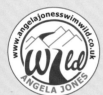

My Adventure Business: Angela Jones Swim Wild and co-founder Jack

Do a job you love and you will never work a day in your life: how true for us both!!!

*Jack would come to work with me everyday and has always been captain of the kayak !!

*Jack has a way of making everyone feel at ease and on wild swims with clients, he picks up on feelings of apprehension so would always swim closer to these clients, making them feel more calm.

*Wild camps were a particular favourite of Jack's. He would never bark at or chase wildlife, allowing clients to embrace nocturnal Nature.

Our beloved business: Jack and I set up together - Swim Wild, Run Wild - has grown steadily and healthily over the last 10 years as Jack and I share our passion and our mission to protect the environment we so dearly love.

I have taken part in several national TV documentaries, contributed to global media articles, and been encouraged to develop commercially as my popularity increases.

Money doesn't drive us, but promoting and spreading the word about our beautiful countryside and protecting and respecting this invitation by Nature does.

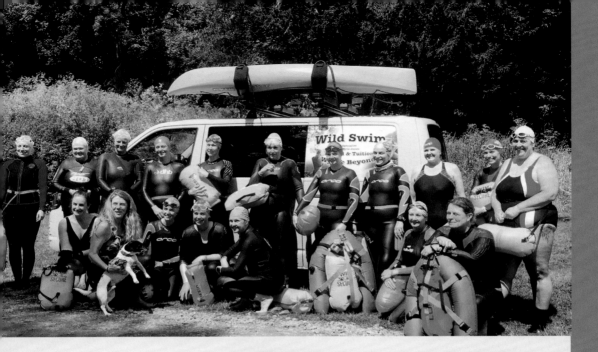

I believe in collaboration rather than competition and encourage people to collaborate with Nature as well as with each other. Of course, enjoyment is important, with confidence boosting being a beautiful by-product.

But safety is paramount. Nature provides us with everything we need to learn, be well and have fun, but she can send in some hefty bills if we are not respectful.

I'm highly qualified, experienced and conscientious in all that I do, including wild swimming.

My wild swimming guidelines also overlap into life skills, as I focus on improving

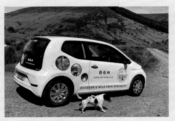

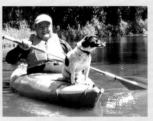

confidence, a positive mindset, enjoyment, motivation, technique and achieving tangible progress. Life, in and out of the water, should be enjoyable and enable personal growth.

And mine and Jack's rewards were knowing that we had shared our inclusive wild side of life with thousands of all ages and abilities over the years.

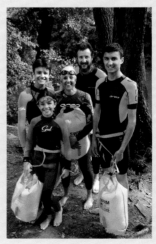

www.angelajonesswimwild.co.uk

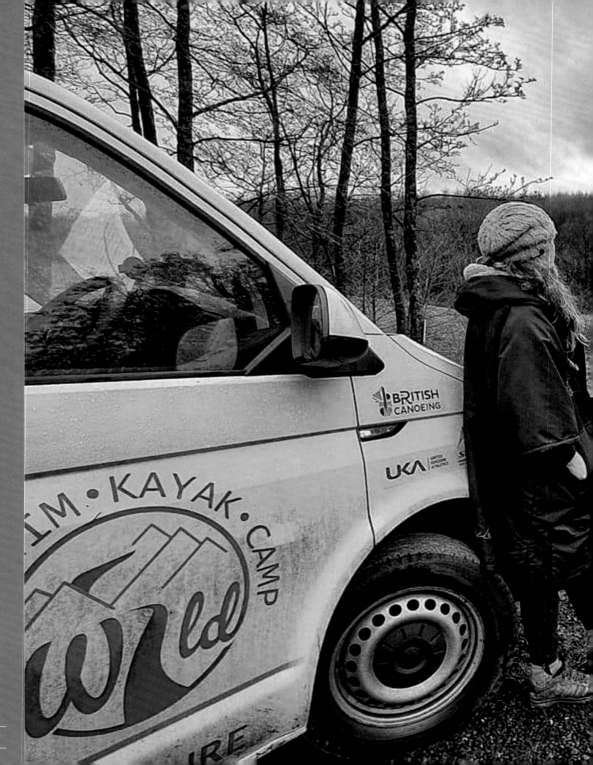

"Swim Wild, Run Wild" has developed organically, from mine and Jack's passion for the wild, dedication to Nature, and our love of the water, in particular, the majestic River Wye."

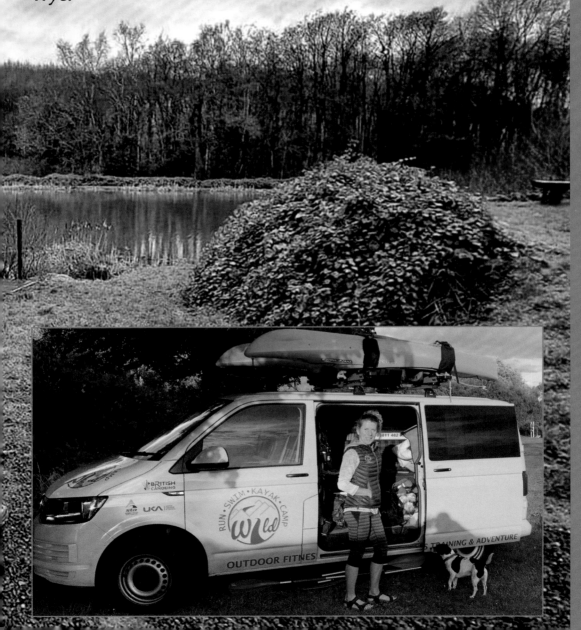

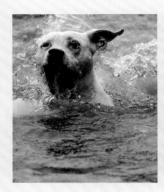
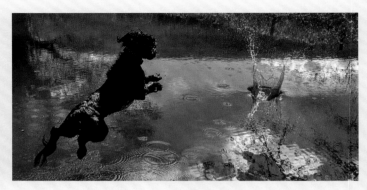

Safety and Rescue

Whilst many people assume that all dogs are born knowing how to swim, that just isn't the case. Every year it is estimated that thousands of family pets drown. And it's not just 'vulnerable' dogs or those in rough oceans and lakes. Drowning happens when a dog becomes completely submerged in water; their lungs are then unable to get oxygen and stop functioning.

Puppies and dogs with short muzzles and barrel chests (e.g., Bulldogs, Pugs) are generally more vulnerable to drowning. This is also true for dogs with cropped or short cork-screwed tails which restrict effective rudder action. This can cause their hind end to sink and result in exhaustion from having to work harder to stay afloat.

Almost all causes of drowning occur due to exhaustion as the dog panics – and the owner too – depleting energy sources quickly.

I've had two tricky occasions – one where my dog got trapped in debris in fast flowing water and another occasion when my dog fell off a 15ft bank into a fast-flowing river. Both times I kept calm and collected and assessed the situation quickly before reacting. I lay down on the riverbank and reached down to assist my dog, being careful not to put myself in danger, to panic or show distress as my dog would have picked up on this. This would have only heightened the danger by putting more fear into the dog.

During the many years I have spent on, in and near rivers, I've witnessed several occasions where owners have panicked and jumped in for their dogs, and every time the dog has got out on their own.

Whenever walking your dog in areas near any bodies of water – like a river, lake, canal or loch – it's important to follow safety guidelines to keep your furry friend safe. Remember, the wet riverbanks, steep edges or jagged rocks can make it hard for a dog to scramble out. These can also be a slip risk for owners. Don't lean into water and try and lift your dog out; you could topple in. And be aware that dogs can experience cold water shock too, which can bring added risks to their health.
If your dog has struggled in the water, it may have inhaled water and should see a vet immediately. Dogs can drown after the event if water has entered their lungs.

CPR Hand Positions

Very small dogs

Medium-Large dogs

Deep-chested dogs

Barrel or flat-chested dogs

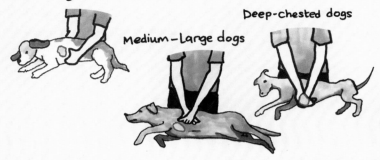
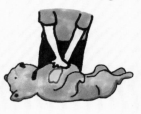

30 Compressions

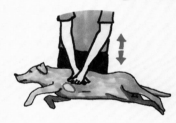
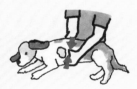

Two breaths

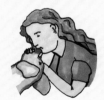

** All dog Parents should Learn CPR for dogs

It is your responsibility as dog parents to learn how to perform CPR on your pet – or indeed anyone else's that you could assist.

Acting calmly, cover your pet's nose with your mouth and exhale until you see the pet's chest rise.

Give a second rescue breath. Continue giving CPR with a cycle of 30 chest compressions and 2 rescue breaths until your dog or cat begins breathing again on its own.

Attending an appropriate course will give you the

knowledge and confidence to act quickly and competently should you need to, and is far better than making an actual 'riverside rescue' your first attempt.

Dry Drowning

Dogs can also suffer from 'near-drowning' or 'dry drowning'. This occurs when water gets into your dog's lungs, or other parts of the airways, while swimming, jumping into the water, or even playing in the bathtub.

It can happen very quickly from merely swallowing a big gulp of water at once.

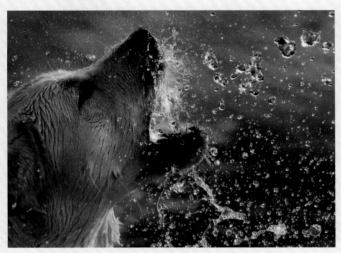

The ingested water can get 'trapped' at the back of the throat and irritate the vocal cords, causing them to spasm. When this occurs, breathing becomes difficult and your dog is likely to panic. When the ingested water enters the lungs, serious complications, and potentially death, can occur.
It is important to know that dry drowning can also occur from swallowing sand whilst your dog plays on the beach. Dogs can show signs of dry drowning hours or even days after the water (or sand) has entered the lungs.
Symptoms of Dry Drowning include:
Coughing   Wheezing
Difficulty breathing   Anxiety
Lethargy, often extreme   Bluish-coloured gums and skin
Discomfort noted, especially around the chest area
Seek veterinary care immediately if you suspect your dog is suffering from dry drowning. With prompt and appropriate treatment, most dogs have a good outcome. If left untreated, dry drowning can be life-threatening.

How to Save a Drowning Dog

Dogs are naturally good swimmers for short distances, but they can get into trouble. Sometimes they get too far from the shore and tire trying to swim back, or they fall into a river and cannot get up the steep sides.

Always protect yourself when trying to rescue a drowning dog. An extra few moments of preparation can save two lives – yours and the dog's. Also be sure to watch for signs of shock, which include pale or white gums, a rapid heartbeat, or rapid breathing.

Useful tips when rescuing a drowning dog.

Rescue the dog.
1: Holding the attached rope, throw a life preserver toward the dog. Make yourself more stable; lower your centre of gravity so you don't topple in.

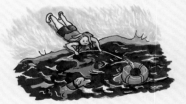

or: 2. Try to hook the dog's collar with a pole.
or: 3. Row out to the dog in a boat.

As a very very last resort, swim to the dog **ONLY** if it's safe to do so. Always protect yourself. Bring something for the dog to cling to or climb on and be pulled to shore.

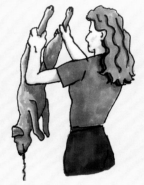

4: Drain the dog's lungs.

5: If you can lift the dog, grasp the rear legs and hold the animal upside down for 15 to 20 seconds. Give 3 or 4 downward shakes to help drain fluid from its lungs.

6: If you cannot lift the dog, place it on a sloping surface with its head low to facilitate drainage.

7: If the dog is not breathing, feel for a heartbeat by placing your fingers about 2 inches behind the dog's elbow in the middle of its chest.

8: If the heart is not beating, perform CPR Use your fingers for smaller dogs and puppies, and your palms for larger dogs. *(see page 77)*

"It's crucial as a pet parent to attend an appropriate Pet First Aid course"

FINALLY, ALWAYS take your dog immediately to the vet. CPR or artificial respiration should be continued until the dog is breathing and its heart is beating without assistance.

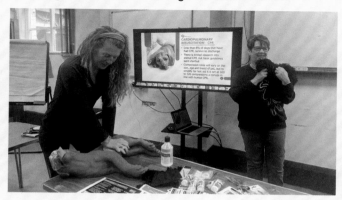

It's crucial as a pet parent to attend an appropriate Pet First Aid course

Water Intoxication

This is caused by drinking, or taking in, too much water into the stomach and occurs when a dog consumes a lot of water in a short amount of time. This causes an electrolyte imbalance within the cells.

The initial symptoms of water intoxication include vomiting, lethargy, and abdominal distention (a bloated belly).

While it sounds crazy that a dog can suffer from the ingestion of too much water, it can happen. This condition is different from dry drowning, which is water (or sand) going into the lungs.

These can progress to include weakness, a lack of co-ordination, seizures, coma and possible death. Treatment by a veterinarian needs to happen as soon as possible. Leaving a dog untreated can be very dangerous. Remember you are your dog's guardian.

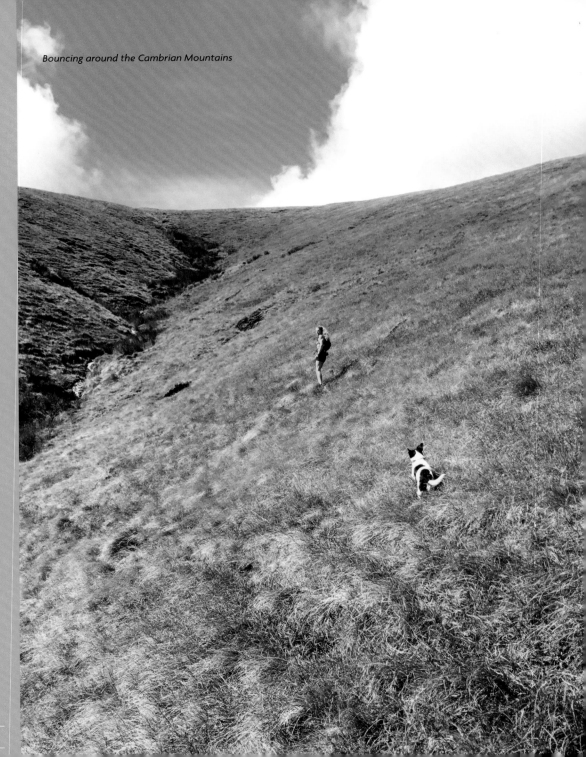

Bouncing around the Cambrian Mountains

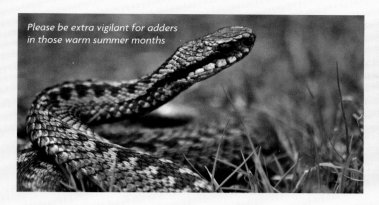
Please be extra vigilant for adders in those warm summer months

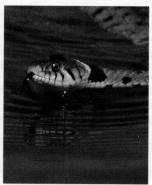

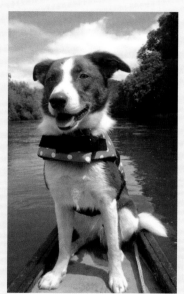

Adder bites

I've had the pleasure of sharing the land and water with several adders over the years. They are shy, beautiful creatures and it's always a pleasure to swim with them – respectfully.

Sadly, this poor Welsh sheep dog called Vilberie didn't survive after being bitten on the face by an adder.

Adders can be found all over the UK and like open habitats such as heathland, moorland, open woodland and sea cliffs. They typically bask on free-draining soils such as chalk or sand and can pose a big threat to our dogs. Puppies and young dogs can be especially curious and an unwelcome investigation can unintentionally provoke an adder into biting. The majority of bites in dogs seem to occur between April and July, most commonly in the afternoon when the adders are most active.

During the many adventures I've been on with my dog, I've come across a good few adders. I've even been bitten whilst out running and it's definitely not a pleasant experience, but like everything in life, it's best not to panic. Try to stay calm and slow down your circulation and heart rate.

Unfortunately, there are many reports of dogs being bitten and sadly not all make it. The best course of action is to take your dog to a vet immediately. If possible, you should carry your dog as this will help to prevent the venom from circulating further around their body. Keep your dog warm and as calm and still as possible, which will also prevent the venom from spreading.

Jean Morris, a vet for over six decades, confirms that adders pose a big threat to our four-legged friends, with over half of adder bites being fatal. So please take extra care and be extra vigilant in those warm summer months.

Water Hazards for your Dog

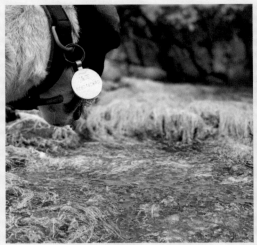

Even on the beach murky pools of seaweed can be harmful to your dog

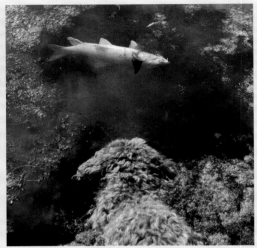

Our local river swim spot in summer often became too toxic to swim: knowing the signs to keeping your woof and you safe is crucial.

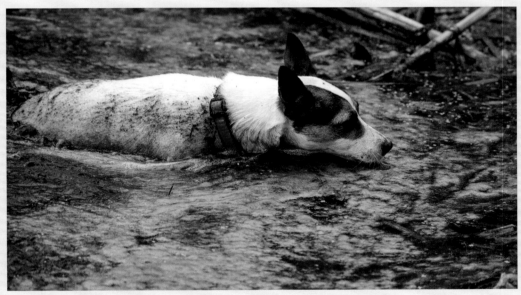

Blue-green algae, or cyanobacteria, is a group of bacteria that can contain dangerous toxins which can be harmful and potentially fatal to pets, livestock and birds if ingested, even in small quantities.

Toxic Blue/ green algae

Please take the time to familiarise yourself with the often hidden dangers posed by 'murky water' that could pose a risk to your dog.

Make sure your dog is up-to-date on their lepto vaccine" Whenever you see a pool of cloudy, stagnant water, your first thought may be 'ugh, gross!' and you'll avoid it but

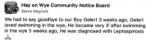

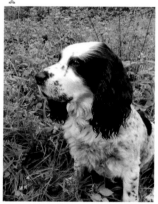

when your dog sees one, they are likely to be deciding which to do first – splash around in it or gulp it down to cool off. Both have the potential to make your dog (and possibly you) very sick.

Diseases such as Leptospirosis and Giardia can be spread to dogs through contaminated water – and passed on to you or a family member. Always make sure your dog is up-to-date on their 'lepto' vaccine to minimise the risk. Unfortunately, there is no vaccine for Giardia, so try to keep your dog away from any still or murky water. Prevention is always better than cure – and whilst you may be seen as 'the bad guy' for spoiling their fun – you may also be saving them a visit to the vet. If you see signs of stomach upset, including particularly foul-smelling diarrhoea, a trip to the vet will be in order.

As a pet parent one of the many water hazards to watch out for is blue-green algae, which is sadly on the increase over the last few years and which can be extremely toxic to dogs. Before heading out on an adventure in a lake or river, I always visually check the water and have learnt over the years how to identify the different algae. I take my water testing kit to be extra safe; testing only takes 15 minutes but can give you peace of mind. I also check local Agency reports for news of any reports of algae blooms. Unfortunately, and very sadly, I know of dogs that have died from polluted waters.
Signs of algae poisoning in dogs include difficulty breathing, muscle weakness, lethargy, and seizures. If you notice these, or any other unusual symptoms after a trip to the water, contact your vet immediately as speedy treatment is critical. And your vet's telephone number should always be in your phone!

While most algae are harmless, some species of blue-green algae produce toxins that can kill a dog within minutes. Dogs that survive (whch are often exposed to low levels of toxins) may develop health problems such as chronic liver disease and possibly tumours - damage that may go unnoticed until it's severe.

Researchers suspect many deaths are deemed 'unexplained' because people don't even realise their dogs were exposed to the algae. Vets may not even recognise the symptoms, and tests to detect the toxins can be costly and complex. It is worth noting that blue-green algae can be harmful to humans too.

IDENTIFYING A HARMFUL ALGAL BLOOM (HAB)

This quick guide provides a visual comparison of appearance, colour and odour that can be helpful in distinguishing non-toxic green algae and aquatic plants from potentially toxic cyanobacteria blooms or harmful algal blooms (HABs).

Non-toxic Algae & Plants   Cyanobacteria/HAB

APPEARANCE

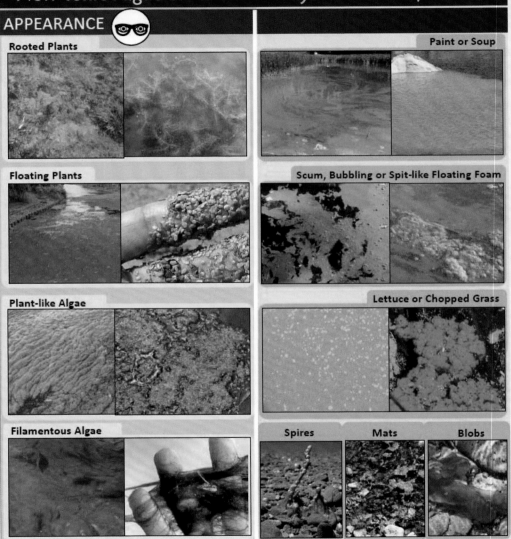

Rooted Plants

Paint or Soup

Floating Plants

Scum, Bubbling or Spit-like Floating Foam

Plant-like Algae

Lettuce or Chopped Grass

Filamentous Algae

Spires   **Mats**   **Blobs**

Even when blue-green algae isn't floating on the surface and visible, it may be lurking below, and will rise and fall with available light and nutrients. At night, it often floats to the top, forming a highly visible scum. Wind and waves can then move and concentrate these toxic blooms in shallow areas or at the water's edge – the places where dogs like to drink and splash about.

Remember a dog just wants to do what dogs do and to have fun – it is your responsibility to make sure that fun is safe.

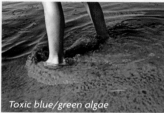
Toxic blue/green algae

The Stick Test

If the stick comes out looking like it has been dipped into a can of paint, the material is likely blue-green algae. If it comes out with long, green, hair-like strands or threads, the material is probably true algae (filamentous green algae).

Here I'm doing the stick test with plant-like algae that is perfectly safe.

Leptospirosis and Giardia

"Make sure your dog is up-to-date on their lepto vaccine"

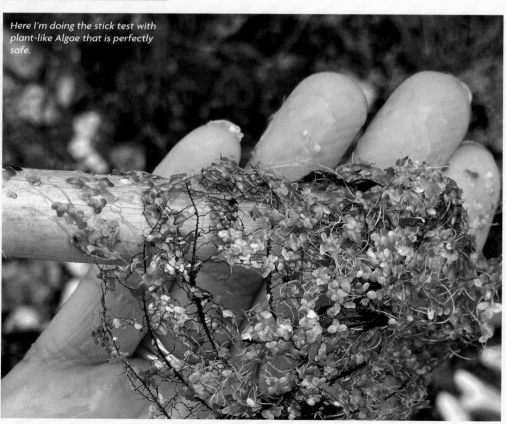
Here I'm doing the stick test with plant-like Algae that is perfectly safe.

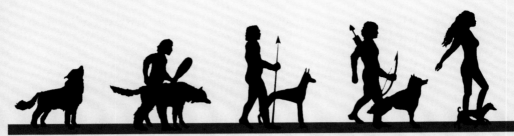

History of dogs

Throughout history, animals have played a key role in human life. People have come to depend on animals for food, clothing, and transportation. At many times throughout history, and in many cultures around the world, animals were also the focus of religious worship.

Although animals still maintain many of those traditional uses around the world, the role of animals in society has also changed. In the last several hundred years, there has been a massive increase in the number of animals kept purely for companionship and pleasure.

Prehistoric communities

The first animal to make the transition from the wild to the domesticated state was the wolf, the common ancestor of all modern-day dogs. This occurred at least 12,000–14,000 years ago when people discovered that young wolf cubs that remained subordinate to humans as adults could be trained. From the earliest days of domestication, dogs would have had practical uses. They were kept because they could perform tasks such as hunting, guarding, and herding. Although domesticated dogs were probably treated with respect in primitive societies, there is evidence that at least some were also considered companions as early as 12,000 years ago. The finding of a Palaeolithic tomb in Northern Israel, in which a human was buried with a dog or wolf puppy, illustrates this point. The dead person's hand had been arranged so that it rested on the animal's shoulder, as if to emphasise a deep bond of affection during life.

Ancient civilisations

A gradual change in human living, from nomadic hunter to settled farmer, began approximately 8,000 years ago in the so-called Fertile Crescent of the Middle East. Working dogs would have been increasingly valued in this setting, but at about this time the cat also became loosely associated with humans. Houses, barns, and grain stores provided a new environmental niche that was rapidly exploited by mice and other small mammals, the favoured prey of small wild felids. Cats that followed these rodents into human settlements would have been tolerated – and possibly encouraged – because of their usefulness in getting rid of these troublesome pests. In some ancient civilisations, dogs may also have had cultural significance, usually in regard to the rise of pet keeping.

This allowed a visible demonstration of man's domination over Nature.

Britain had been a centre for dog breeding since Roman times, and one of the first formal competitive dog shows was held in Newcastle in 1859 for the Pointer and Setter breeds. Still, little was known about the inheritance of various characteristics until Charles Darwin published *The Origin of the Species* in 1859. Since that time, dog breeding has become more formalised with the establishment of strict breed standards.

The practice of pet keeping in Victorian times also reflected other social attitudes of the time. Pet keeping was not considered appropriate for the 'lower classes,' as it was thought to encourage the neglect of other social duties.

Pet keeping in modern society

In present-day societies, dogs have a number of functional roles, from ornamental to status symbol; as helpers, and as companions. Dogs can also act as a channel for personal expression because people express their personality in the breed they own. For example, rare breeds are often used as indicators of status. Guide dogs for blind people and hearing dogs for deaf people are examples of pets that are kept as helpers.

But the most common reason for owning pets in Western societies is companionship. In recent years, there's been a growing awareness of the very positive effects this relationship can have on human health and psychological well-being, and a recognition of the therapeutic value of companion animals.

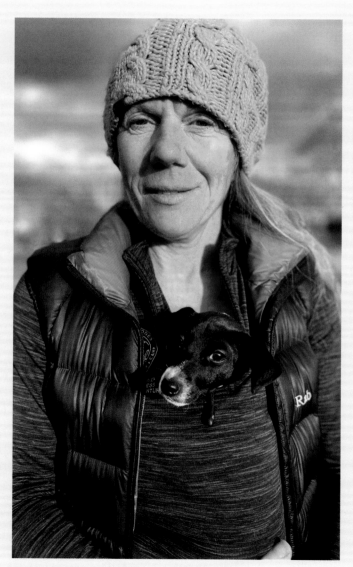

Bonding with Junior, on his first day.

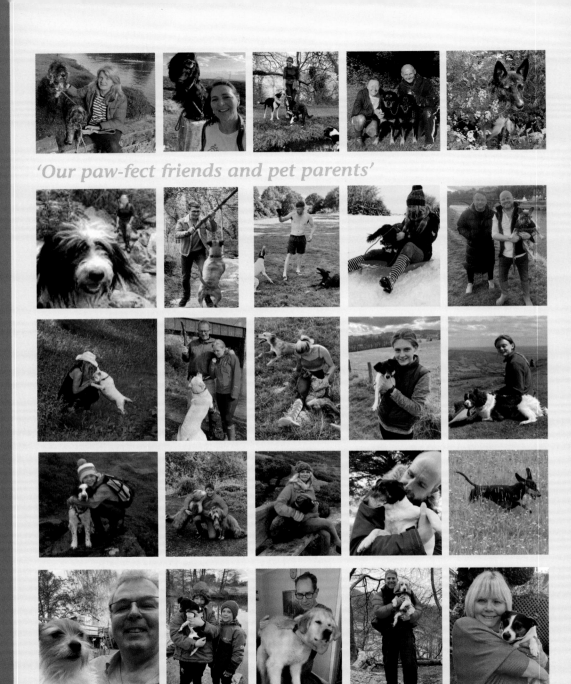

'Our paw-fect friends and pet parents'

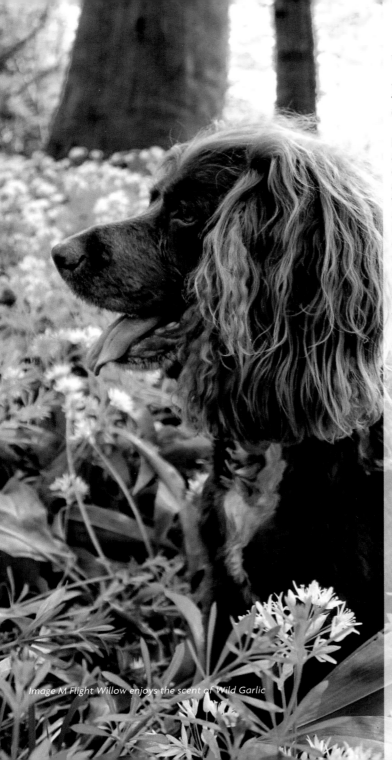

You can't fool your dog's sense of smell

Research indicates that a dog's sense of smell can pick up fear, anxiety and even sadness. The flight-or-fight hormone, adrenaline, is undetectable by our noses, but dogs can apparently smell it. In addition, fear or anxiety is often accompanied by increased heart rate and blood flow, which sends tell-tale body chemicals more quickly to the skin surface. Trying to mask your strong feelings with a casual smile may fool your friends, but it's not going to fool a dog's sense of smell.

Image M Flight Willow enjoys the scent of Wild Garlic

Scientists report a dog's sense of smell is 10,000 - 100,000 times more acute than humans.

Snacks in the wild - activity and reward

Hide your dog's homemade treats on your adventure walks and in woodlands and see how much extra pleasure your woof gets from searching and finding them.
Dogs love to use their imagination. It's second nature to them. While they're working, they're gaining skills and strength and having fun.

They're enjoying physical and mental stimulation which all in all makes for a happier, healthier dog. And if there's a treat as a reward at the end of it, your best friend is simply going to love you all the more!

Level 1
Starting out low land activity treats ideal for building up strength and agility.

Level 2
Advanced balancing and technical agility for building up core and co-ordination.

Depending on size and breed these adventure treat sessions should be adapted to suit your dog.

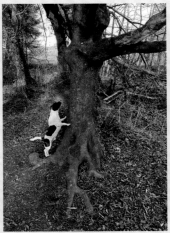

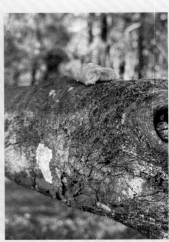

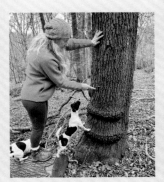

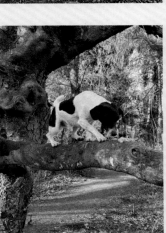

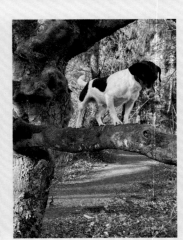

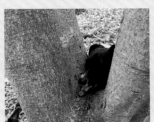

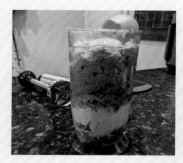

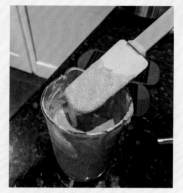

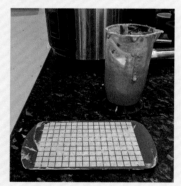

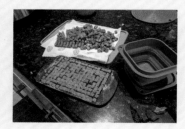

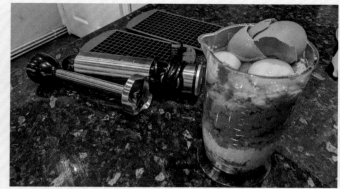

Making your own doggy treats

200g fish/meat
4 heaped tbsp of flour – oat, buckwheat, rice, wholewheat, etc.
1 egg – can include shell
Fruit/veggies/herbs/spices
1 tsp coconut oil

photos are Forthglade 90% chicken liver, spelt flour, egg, cooked carrot, cooked broccoli, cheese, rocket, fresh ginger, turmeric, coconut oil.

1. Add your ingredients and blend thoroughly.
2. The consistency should be thick but still possible to pour and spread. Add more flour if it is too runny; add some water or other liquid if it is too thick. The consistency will change depending on how much liquid is in your meat/ fish, fruit and veggies.
3. Spread the paste across a silicone mould – mini ice cube ones work well, or pyramid pans.
4. For mini ice cube trays, cook in the microwave for 5 mins or the oven for 20-30 mins. Adjust the time depending on how squidgy (less time) or crunchy (more time) you want the treats, and for the size of mould.
5. The treats should easily pop out of the mould: if they are getting stuck then you may need to cook them for a little longer.

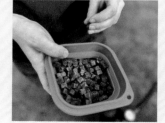

Dog Food

I've learnt a lot about the appropriate food to give my dog and puppy whilst out on our adventures and am sharing it so you don't have to learn by your mistakes!

It is best to avoid taking foil pouches of wet dog food on any adventure. Despite being convenient in some respects, temperature changes can drastically and catastrophically change the contents, which in turn can prove a real risk to your dog's health and wellbeing.

One of our day-long hikes ended with an emergency dash to the vet. Whilst hiking, I decided to give my dog an afternoon treat of a meaty dog food pouch, only to find him fall very ill rapidly. We quickly descended the mountain and I rushed him to the emergency vets, who diagnosed food poisoning. It was an awful time and was touch and go for a few days, causing us both a huge amount of stress. By sharing this experience with you I can save you and your four-legged friend the same distress.

Similarly, avoid storing the dog food pouches in the car or anywhere the temperature could change significantly – it happens more than you think. Please be 'pouch-aware' when it comes to your pooch!

Dried food is the best option for your joint adventures. I take additional carrots, cucumber, apple, nuts, and rice cakes – four-leggeds and two-leggeds can share these treats! And just like us, dogs get sugar rushes if they snack on sugary stuff, and after the rushes will come lows – which are not good for you or your canine companion. Energy supplies always need to be consistent and like tending a fire, best results are achieved by constant monitoring and regular feeding – especially whilst out on adventures where energy can be burned quicker.

Also hiking and having a scone for lunch I accidentally dropped a piece, containing currents, which my dog wafted up: again one very sick dog and a worried owner !

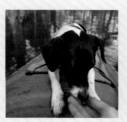

Junior enjoys a snack on his kayaking trip.

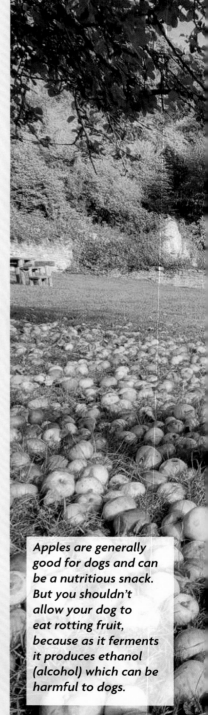

Apples are generally good for dogs and can be a nutritious snack. But you shouldn't allow your dog to eat rotting fruit, because as it ferments it produces ethanol (alcohol) which can be harmful to dogs.

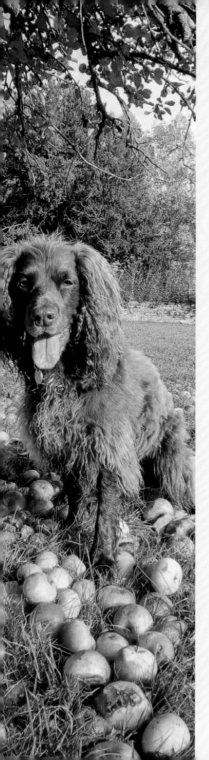

Vegetables and fruits are great for deworming dogs. They contain high levels of fibre which help to bulk up the stools and expel the worms. Pumpkin, carrots, sweet potatoes, apples, and papaya are all excellent choices. Feeding your dog a couple of these a day will help to clean them out and keep them healthy.

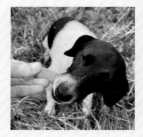

Foods and items that are poisonous to dogs:

Drugs: Prescription drugs that might be beneficial or even lifesaving for people can have the opposite effect on pets – and it doesn't take a large dose to do major damage. Always keep your dog away from prescription drugs – and remember that some dogs will eagerly explore your bag. I have heard horror stories of dogs that have found and eaten Paracetamol and other over-the-counter drugs that they found in a bag. Sadly, sometimes you may not even know that the dog has taken the drugs – until they are poorly. Please be responsible around these prescription drugs – dogs don't understand they are not designed for them.

A lot of 'people food' is poisonous to dogs. What we may find delicious can be deadly for our four-legged friends. It may seem unkind not to share a tasty piece of chocolate cake or scone but that 'kindness' could kill.

Animals have different metabolisms than people, and some foods, such as onions and garlic, and even some beverages that are enjoyed by people can be dangerous, and sometimes fatal, for dogs.

Alcohol: Symptoms of alcohol poisoning in animals are similar to those in people, and may include vomiting, breathing problems, slipping into a coma and, in severe cases, death.

Avocado: Considered a healthy addition to human diets, avocados contain a substance called persin that is toxic to dogs, causing vomiting and diarrhoea.

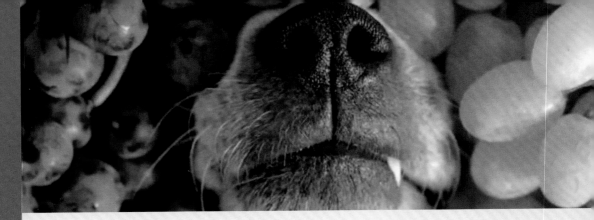

Grapes and raisins: Experts aren't sure why, but these fruits can induce kidney failure in dogs and even a small number may cause problems in some dogs.

Xylitol: This sweetener is found in many products, including sugar-free drinks and sweets. It causes a rapid drop in blood sugar, resulting in weakness and seizures. Liver failure has also been reported in some dogs. Xylitol itself – and sweets – are another example of things that a dog may 'find' in your bag or pocket and 'snaffle' before you realise.

Other foods you should keep away from your pet include tomatoes, mushrooms and most seeds and nuts.

Household products: I think it is best to assume that all household products are dangerous to our pets and therefore keep them all out of harm's way. Just as things like bleach can poison people, they are also a leading cause of pet poisoning, resulting in stomach and respiratory tract problems. Not surprisingly, chemicals contained in antifreeze, paint thinners, and chemicals for pools and gardens are often toxic to dogs – and children – and therefore should always be kept safely stored away from both!

The 'icides': Rodenticides, pesticides and insecticides all contain chemicals that can harm your dog and at worst prove fatal. Unfortunately, many baits used to lure and kill rodents can also 'lure' our pets. If ingested by dogs, they can cause severe problems. The symptoms depend on the nature of the poison, and signs may not start for several days after consumption – which is often not witnessed. In some instances, the dog may have eaten the poisoned rodent, and although not been directly exposed to the toxin, can still suffer dire consequences.

Insecticides such as bug sprays and ant baits are often kept on shelves in sheds and can be easy for your pet to get into. They are as dangerous for your pet as they are to the insects.

If you think your dog has been poisoned, try to stay calm. It is important to act quickly, but rationally. Panicking never helps anything.
First, gather up any of the

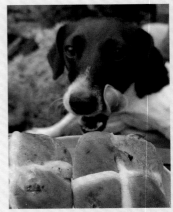

Out hiking and having a scone for lunch I accidentally dropped a piece, containing currants, which my dog hoovered up: one very sick dog and a worried owner!

What to do for suspected dog poisoning

potential poison that remains if you can (even chocolate wrappers as they will have the ingredients listed) as this may be helpful to your vet and any outside experts who assist with the case. If your dog has already vomited, collect the sample in case your veterinarian needs to see it. As a responsible paw-rent, you must be aware of the risks to your dogs – educate yourself about the potential dangers and share your knowledge with others. There is no need to be neurotic about it but prevention is ALWAYS better than cure.

NEVER take wet dog food out on adventures or keep in rucksack or vehicle as temperature changes can result in various ingredients becoming toxic and therefore being extremely dangerous to your dog. I found this out the hard way by having to rush my dog to emergency vets. This is why I urge you to share knowledge and experiences.

Accidents will happen which is why it is important to know what to do in the event.

Even some plants can be toxic to dogs and whilst many dogs won't be tempted by them, some are just inquisitive and want to know what they taste

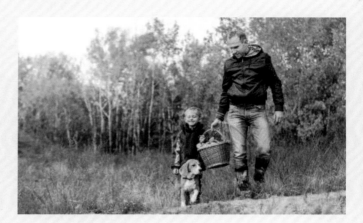

like. Always try to 'watch' your dog. It irks me to see people on their mobile phones whilst walking their four-legged friends. You will miss far more interesting things than you will ever see on your phone as well as keeping a caring eye on your pooch.

The most obvious way to know that your pet has eaten a dangerous plant, is to catch them in the act. Once spotted, call your vet for advice straight away – don't wait for symptoms to appear.

Our pets are curious by nature and at times may be tempted to lick or chew plants and trees. Sadly, not everything they explore in this way is harmless, and Nature has her own way of protecting herself, so it's important to know which plants could potentially cause problems – for humans as well as for dogs.

Owners must always be aware that there are poisonous plant and fungal species that exist in the wild. Nature is not all about pretty flowers and fluffy clouds. Given the difficulty in identifying which species a dog may come across, all mushroom ingestions should be treated as emergencies by owners and veterinarians alike.

As a general rule, try your best to keep your dog away from mysterious mushrooms growing outdoors.

5 Reasons Dog Owners Must SCOOP THAT POOP

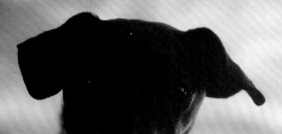

1. Dog poop is classified as a pollutant, not fertilizer - it destroys ecosystems.

2. Some dog poop contains harmful organisms such as E. coli and parasitic worms.

3. Rain washes dog poop into water systems, infiltrating drinking and swimming water and harming aquatic life

4. Dog poop creates a hazard for other animals as well as humans.

5. It is a dog owner's responsibility to clean up after their pet.

Let's talk CR*P

Studies show that roughly 40% of all dog owners do not 'stoop and scoop'. Don't kid yourself – the ecosystem doesn't gracefully embrace dog waste. If left intact, it can take more than a year to break down and can quickly, and selfishly, turn any outdoor area into a site unfit for pets and humans.

In addition to the mess and smell, raw dog waste kills grass and plants and encourages noxious weed infestations. Residual waste left at ground zero runs off untreated into storm sewers and waterways. You may think, "If it's OK for a bear to poo in the woods, why not dogs?" This is why...

Recent studies indicate that dogs are third or fourth on the list of contributors to bacteria in contaminated waters, increasing the potential for serious diseases, including cholera and dysentery. The EPA estimates that two days' worth of dog waste from about 100 dogs can create enough pollution to close a bay and all the watersheds within 20 miles.

In addition to threats to humans, bacteria that feed on dog waste deplete oxygen, killing native aquatic life. The bacteria also feed algae blooms that block sunlight and suffocate fish. Dog waste toxins themselves can significantly increase fish mortality. There is a tendency to assume that since bears, sheep, horses, deer and other wild animals poop in the woods, it's OK for our dogs to do the same. But before you walk away from your pal's latest deposit into the ecosystem, please think again.

Dog waste is far more harmful to water, land and air than you might think and a quick 'stoop and scoop' can make all the difference to our wildlife and our environment.

Last resort, if you are camping in a remote area deposit pet waste in a 6-8" deep hole at least 200 feet (70 big steps) away from any water sources to avoid contamination.

Many studies have shown that compostible poo bags will not biodegrade in the natural environment. They remain intact for years before fragmenting into micro plastics.
Dr Alice Judge, January 2024

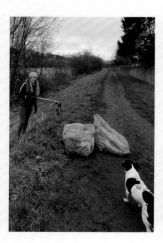

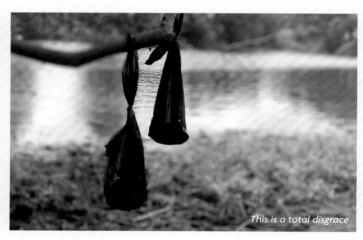

This is a total disgrace

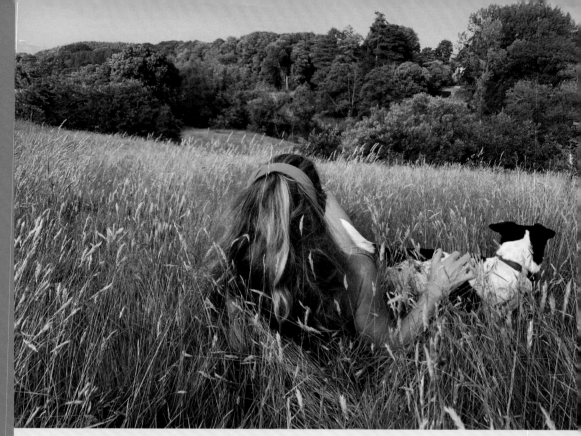

Jack and I love being amongst Grasslands — unfortunately the prime habitat for ticks and fleas; but with vigilance and care, there are precautions we can take to minimise the risks.

How to identify ticks

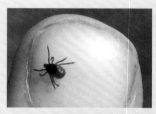

There are three types of tick commonly found in the UK: *Ixodes ricinus* (the sheep/deer tick); *Ixodes hexagonus* (the hedgehog tick) and *Ixodes canisuga* (the British dog or fox tick). Ticks can live for up to three years and will feed on the blood of a single host in each of their life stages — as larvae, nymphs and adults. While living on their host, they will also find a mate with which they will reproduce.

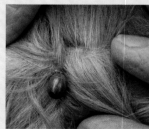

Before they have fed on the blood of their host, ticks are so tiny they can be mistaken for a speck of dirt or a poppy seed. A tick remains attached to their host for approximately five days while feeding. After feeding, adult ticks become lighter in colour and can be the size of a small pea. Although we usually associate ticks with warm summers and lush, long grass, their numbers are rising across the UK as a result of changing climates and habitats, and an increasing number of hosts.

Ticks are so small that they can be mistaken for a freckle, but they can cause Lyme disease, which affects both humans and animals and can be fatal in the worst cases.

Where are ticks found?

Ticks usually live in woodland and heath areas, and like warmer and wetter weather conditions. The increase in wild deer numbers has also contributed to a rise in the number of ticks, as they like to live on the skin of wild deer.

Where are fleas found?

In your garden and in wildlife, fleas live in high grass, sand, sheds and débris – places where they can find shade and humidity. These areas, such as the grass underneath shrubs, provide the perfect conditions for all three stages of the flea's life cycle.

The places we frequent with our dogs during adventures or whilst walking, commonly have heather, bracken, grassland or woodland. These are generally prime habitat for ticks and fleas but with vigilance and care, there are precautions we can take to minimise the risks, such as covering up bare skin and using environmentally-friendly repellent(for yourself not your dog). It is so important to check your woof and yourself after every walk adventure as I'm only too aware, as both myself and Jack have had extra unwanted passengers over the years!

I have written to UK vets and suppliers of spot-on treatments to bring awareness so that these highly hazardous chemicals are taken off sale.

In recent years we have been focussing on the impact that farming has on the environment with the use of chemicals, antibiotics, and anthelmintics (worming treatments) under scrutiny. So it is only natural that our thoughts should turn to animals closer to home too. The advice has always been to use regular preventative parasite treatment on our pets to protect the health of that individual. But what impact might this be having on the environment?

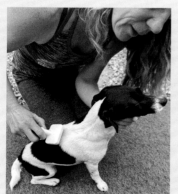

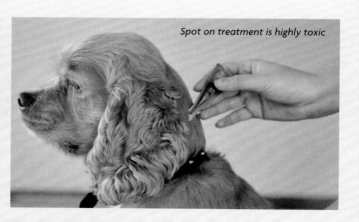

Spot on treatment is highly toxic

Preventing fleas from infesting dogs

Check dogs for fleas by using a flea comb after hiking in the woods or walking in tall grass.

Prevention is the best way to keep dogs safe from fleas. Dogs will not get fleas if pet parents pay attention and follow several appropriate steps.

• Use natural flea prevention sprays or essential oils to deter fleas from leaping onto your dog.

• Use a flea comb and brush the dog's coat after every walk. Check for signs of fleas or ticks and remove them immediately.

• Brush the dog's coat regularly. Brushing the coat is good for skin health, promotes bonding, and allows owners to check the skin for fleas at the end of the day.

• Buy and use natural flea collars that have essential oil scents or sound-modulating technology to deter fleas and ticks.

Are tick and flea treatments a problem?

Recently there have been questions raised as to the impact that flea and tick treatment has on environmental contamination and insect populations. After all, tick and flea treatment is insecticidal, which is how it does its job of killing ticks and fleas (a wingless insect parasite). These products affect other insects and invertebrate populations too, causing devastation to eco-systems.

Recent studies show alarming levels of two chemicals, fipronil and imidacloprid, in rivers and lakes which is extremely worrying.

Concentrations of these chemicals are particularly high just downstream of waterworks, suggesting that these chemicals are coming down sewers through treated pets being bathed at home, and through inappropriate disposal of these products too.

Fipronil is a product readily available to the general public as an over-the-counter flea medication, with no veterinary prescription required. This means it is probably one of the most common flea products used.

What could be done about it?

One idea proposed is to tighten regulations and make this drug prescription only to help manage its use more appropriately. Another idea is to consider using targeted parasite products rather than using these chemicals prophylactically all year round. This does have the downside that your pet would not be protected against parasites all year round, and would have to catch them before treatment can be implemented. This idea is sound in theory, but having seen the real difficulty that some owners face when trying to get rid of a full-blown flea infestation, it's hard to see that we could legitimately go back to this. Most owners are now very diligent at ensuring their pet's preventative parasite treatment is up to speed and the health of our pets is foremost in our minds. So instead of not treating pets at all, perhaps we should look at some of the individual products we are using instead?

Collars and environmental impacts

Flea and tick collars can often be purchased without a veterinary prescription. Some of these collars can last several months, which provides ongoing protection even in the face of forgetful owners! Some collars are water-resistant and so can be worn whilst swimming or being bathed. However, one popular product contradicts this by stating 'This product should not enter water courses as it is dangerous to fish and other aquatic organisms'. This raises some environmental questions, especially if you have a dog that spends most of its time swimming.

"One flea treatment of a medium-sized dog with imidacloprid contains enough pesticide to kill 60 million bees and also has a devastating impact on all our water sources."

Spot on products are having a devastating effect on our eco-systems.

Spot-on flea treatments are probably the most common product used on our pet dogs. There are a variety of spot-ons used including, but not limited to, those that contain fipronil and imidacloprid. The advantage of spot-on treatments is that they are 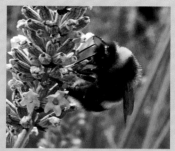 very easy to administer, with an application of a small volume of liquid to the back of the neck once a month (for most products). Many of these products protect against multiple parasites. The disadvantage of spot-ons is that they can get easily washed off. Especially if your dog is bathed or goes swimming, causing devastating impact on ecosystems and waterways.

Tablets

There are different types of flea tablets available for dogs, some of which cover other parasites like ticks too. These tablets are ingested by your pet and protect for up to 3 months in the case of some tablets. The advantage of tablets is that your dog can swim and be bathed without it reducing the efficacy of the product. This is because the molecules are held within your dog's skin, rather than being applied on the surface. Of course, some dogs will refuse to take tablets, which can make life tricky. In the datasheet for one of these tablets the active ingredient, Fluralaner, is stated to be excreted almost unchanged in the faeces, so more devastating impact on the environment. So which is best?

It is best to speak with your veterinary surgeon to balance the individual needs of your dog alongside any environmental concern. Why not use Natural Insect Control and protect your woof and the environment?

What flea treatment for dogs is most environmentally friendly?

Thankfully, there are several natural methods for eliminating the threat of these pests. Specific flower scents and natural sprays are capable of eliminating these insects before they completely infest your home. But PLEASE check that anything you use is NOT harmful to your pet.

Please STOP using harsh chemicals on your dog and try a more natural method for removing fleas from your pooch.

Prevention is the best way to keep dogs safe from fleas. Dogs will not get fleas if pet parents pay attention and follow several appropriate steps.

Methods of removing fleas naturally from dogs

Some medication-sensitive dogs have experienced adverse side effects from modern medications. People are looking for alternative options to toxic chemicals. Thankfully, natural flea and tick remedies are abundant, as humans have been combating these pests for thousands of years.

Natural Flea Sprays

Flea sprays with natural ingredients are gentle and reduce risk of adverse side effects.

Natural flea sprays are chemical-free and found at holistic integrative veterinary clinics and pet stores. These sprays use safe and gentle water-based solvents to safely kill fleas and eggs.

Application

Spray the dog's entire body with natural flea sprays. Then, put on a pair of gloves and brush the dog's coat. The spray is safe for human skin, but the gloves are used to prevent fleas from leaping onto the owner. Massage the solvent into the dog's fur, making sure it reaches the skin and undercoat (if applicable). After waiting the allotted time according to the bottle or veterinarian's instructions, use a flea comb to brush out any remaining dead fleas.

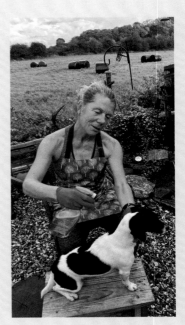

Junior sits patiently – Natural flea sprays protect your woof and the environment we love.

Essential Oils

Many natural essential oils are harmful and toxic to pets whether inhaled, consumed orally or absorbed through the skin so it is essential you research this fully and get professional advice, as social media and websites are full of contradictory information that could lead to a very poorly woof!

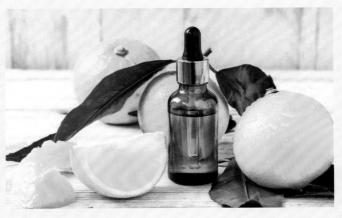

Organic Flea Treatment Shampoos

Organic flea shampoos are a two-fold method of removing fleas from dogs and making them smell fresh and clean. Normal soap and water can kill most fleas, but organic flea shampoos use natural ingredients to target and remove fleas and eggs.

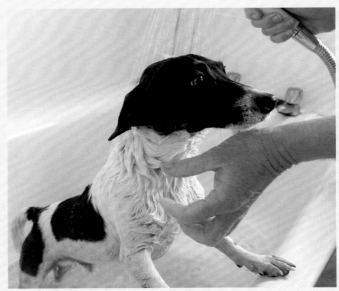

Application

Avoid getting water in the dog's eyes and ears. Too much moisture in the ears will cause ear infections, which will require medical treatment.

Soap and Water

Regular pet-safe soap and water can be used to effectively remove fleas and ticks from the coat.

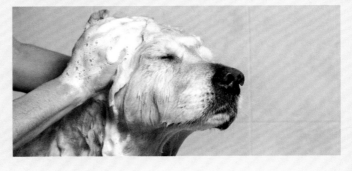

How to make the perfect puppy introduction

Introductions between a puppy and an older dog are far more likely to go smoothly if you set yourself up to succeed by following some top tips.

1. Swap scents

Before picking up your new puppy ask the owner, breeder or shelter manager to provide you with a towel or blanket that's got the pup's scent on it. Scent is very important to a dog.

Letting your older dog smell the puppy's scent ahead of time will get them used to the approaching arrival. Likewise, to help the puppy overcome their first-meeting nerves, give them something with your home scent on beforehand. That way when you meet you won't be completely unfamiliar to them. Get vaccinations up to date.

Just like having appropriate dog insurance, regular vaccinations and check-ups are part of responsible dog ownership. At a young age, puppies are particularly vulnerable to infection. So, it's important your adult dog is fully vaccinated before they meet.

Puppies themselves are typically vaccinated at eight and 10 weeks (although they can be vaccinated as early as between four and six weeks of age) with the second dose usually being given two to four weeks later.

2. Get vaccinations up to date

Vaccinations are usually needed to protect against things like:
- Canine distemper
- Canine parvovirus
- Kennel cough
- Leptospirosis
- Parainfluenza

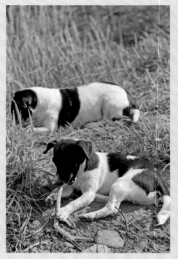

Young Junior lets Jack have his own space !

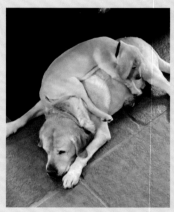

Here my friend's puppy shows his affections to his big bro !!

3. Keep a distance at first meeting

For safety's sake keeping the two dogs apart but allowing them to sniff each other at their first meeting is a good idea. Either through a fence or through the puppy's crate will let them get to know each other's scents and sounds. It also means you'll feel more relaxed, thereby keeping your dogs calm, too.

This is of particular importance when there's a big size difference between the adult dog and the new pup. Unfortunately, even a very friendly adult dog can easily injure the youngster with over-exuberant greetings. Accidents do happen and prevention is always better than cure.

4. Start off on neutral ground

Dogs are very territorial creatures so a first meeting in your adult dog's home territory might create unnecessary problems. It's recommended to introduce them first at a park or in someone else's garden. That way your dog won't feel threatened or protective of their home and might be more willing to accept the new pup.

5. Take some parallel walks together

Take the puppy and older dog for a walk with a family member or friend. It's a great way to allow a meeting in a natural canine social environment.

Allow plenty of nose sniffing but make sure you break it up with lots of walking. The walk will be a great distraction for both dogs, allowing familiarity to build and tension to reduce. Start off on neutral ground.

Furthermore, exploring new smells and sights together is a good way for them to bond. Hopefully, the pup will look to the older dog for reassurance while the older dog will put a protective paw around the youngster.

Warning – Until their vaccinations are complete it's not safe for your puppy to be put on the ground in public places. In the meantime, the puppy should not be allowed to walk anywhere unvaccinated dogs could have been. Having dog insurance in place is important to protect your new pup if anything untoward happens when you're out and about.

6. Play training games

Just as with parallel walks, playing training games is a fun way to keep dogs active but also distracted during early introductions. For your pup, consider taking them to puppy training classes.

Keep any eye on any aggression developing. You don't want all your good work to become undone!

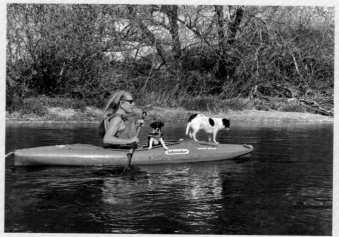

Here Jack teaches the new kid on the block kayaking skills

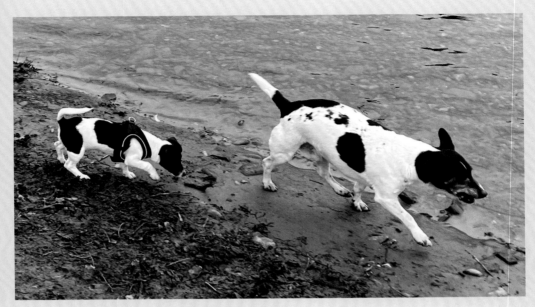

16-week old Junior learns the ropes by following his mentor mature Jack

7. Praise the positive play. The tail end going up and the head going down is a classic canine invitation to some rough and tumble.

If the puppy licks the mouth and face of the older dog and rolls on their back then it's communicating submission. This is a good sign they already understand some of the rules of the dog world.

Whines, barks and growls can be either playful or threatening depending on the circumstances. Always pay attention to any body language suggesting this.

Look out for doggy language that they're happy to play. The tail end going up and the head going down is a classic canine invitation to some rough and tumble.

8. Move to home ground when they're both ready

Once they've got to know each other in neutral areas you can start to move toward home territory. Start off with garden introductions before going inside. It's often better for the resident dog to arrive at the house and find the puppy already there inside.

Body language to watch out for:

For the first week or two, never leave the older dog and puppy alone together, even for a moment. Be sure to follow your older dog's regular routine and also begin establishing a puppy routine. The more consistent you are, the more likely you are to succeed.

Closely observing both dogs' body language for the first few weeks will help you assess how they're getting on. If the puppy is young, it may not yet understand the body language of the adult dog.

For instance, the puppy will likely want to play even if the older dog is showing clear signs of annoyance. Being jumped on, walked on and having their ears and tail nipped is likely to test the patience of even the most chilled-out hound.

Look out for these clear signs that a line has been crossed:

- Raised fur on the back of the neck/back
- Prolonged stares
- Growling
- Snarling
- Display of teeth
- Hunched back

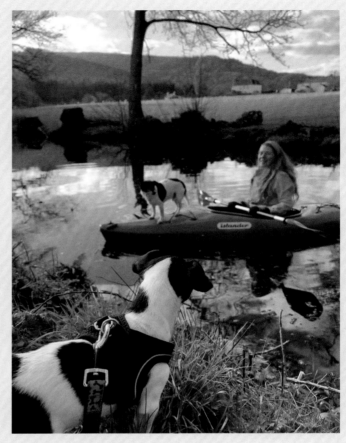

Young Junior is introduced to Jack's adventurous life gently

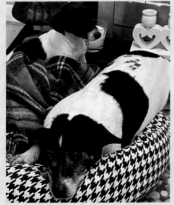

Scent is very important to a dog so sharing puppy's blanket ahead of arrival is very important

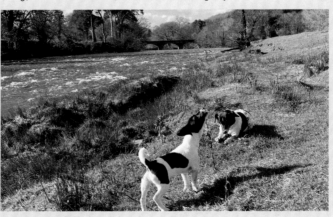

The woeful demise of our wonderful rivers and seas

I have been witnessing and monitoring our rivers, and their relationship with the countryside, closely over the past decades – and especially for the last five years. During that time I have seen a huge increase in farming pollution, slurry discharge, water extraction for irrigating farm fields, contamination from chemical crop sprays and industries, and a catastrophic increase in contamination from raw sewage entering our rivers and seas.

I've also witnessed a huge increase in plastic in our rivers and seas. Coming from businesses, tourists and locals alike, it is both shameful and pitiful to see it clogging up Nature's arteries throughout the UK.

There are many people who care for our rivers but alas, far too many who are just happy to take advantage of them, without a thought for the long and short-term effects on our

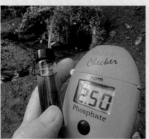
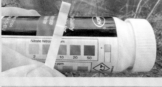
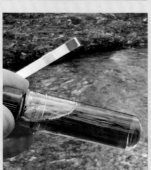
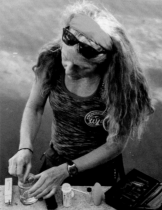

Data is crucial to holding polluters to account. Over the years I've trained up many water testing volunteers and help set up many groups around the country.

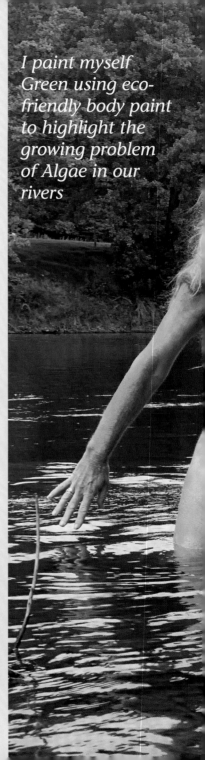

I paint myself Green using eco-friendly body paint to highlight the growing problem of Algae in our rivers

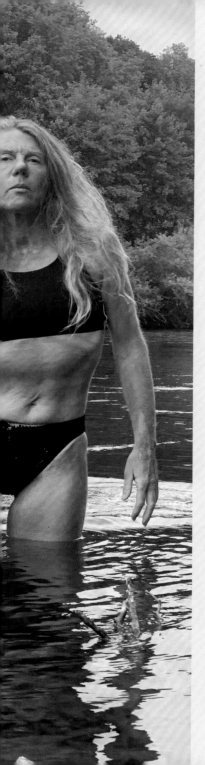

precious waterways - the veins that support the ecological biodiversity of so many species.

Over the past five or six years I have also witnessed an increase in toxic green algae and there are now serious concerns over the permanently damaging effects these severe blooms are having on the ecology of our highly protected rivers — on top of everything else.

Almost all of the UK's waterways are polluted.

In 2022, a House of Commons Committee report on the state of UK rivers concluded that 'no river in UK was free from chemical contamination'. Only 14% of UK rivers had a 'good' ecological status and the sheer volume of pollution in coastal waters has resulted in the UK being ranked one of the worst in Europe.

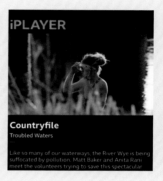

iPLAYER

Countryfile
Troubled Waters

Like so many of our waterways, the River Wye is being suffocated by pollution. Matt Baker and Anita Rani meet the volunteers trying to save this spectacular

I was asked to speak in Westminster in February 2023 to deliver the data and evidence of pollution that I have been collecting first-hand. Since doing so I have been invited back to the Houses of Parliament to contribute to various further discussions and reports.

I have established numerous Citizen Science Water Testing Groups, have given speeches and provided training all over the country in order to share my knowledge and experience. This allows a wider audience to gather the essential data, enabling them to protect their own water space, and also encourages and empowers them to hold the polluters to account.

I utilise my media profile as a springboard to bring awareness to this environmental disaster, which is unfolding in front of our very eyes. I campaign tirelessly, training up volunteers, working with scientists and making

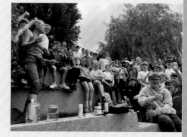

Here I teach schoolchildren how to protect their river.

numerous media and public appearances countrywide.

I have contributed to a BBC *Panorama* documentary, BBC News, *Countryfile*, and many other media projects over the years and I was instrumental in bringing a Bill to Parliament to clean up our rivers – and I will continue to lobby Government to tighten up the law to protect and clean up our rivers and seas – all of which I do voluntarily and without any financial gain.

I generously and enthusiastically share my first-hand knowledge of the pollution caused by raw sewage and agricultural and industrial waste that continues to blight our rivers and seas. And I also take action.

I am not a lone crusader or a crank. I just know what's right – and what's not. And I am prepared to take the actions necessary to raise awareness of the colossal importance of preserving the health of our water and the wildlife it supports – for generations to come.

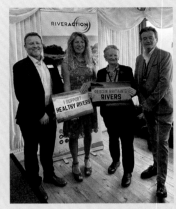

River Action, Campaign launch

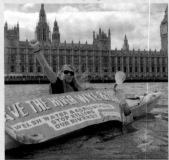

Campaigning outside Westminster

Where it all began: River Wye, Monmouth

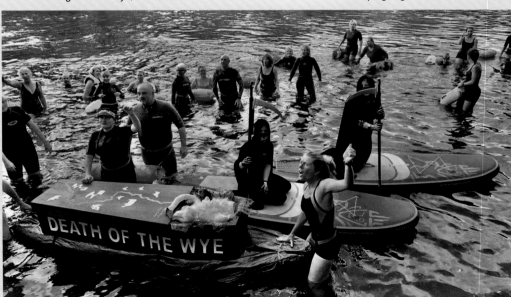

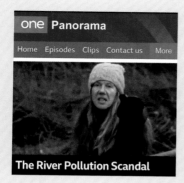

The River Pollution Scandal

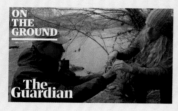

SO HOW CAN YOU HELP?

Please report ANY pollution ASAP. Give time, date and location.

In Wales you can contact Natural Resources Wales on 0300 065 3000 Email: enquiries@naturalresourceswales.gov.uk In England you can contact Natural England by emailing enquiries@naturalengland.org.uk

Or The Environment Agency at 0370 8506506 enquiries@environment-agency.gov.uk

And of course you can contact your local MP and ask for their intended actions.

'There is power in numbers and power in unity. Please don't look the other way "together we can bring that change"

At Hay Festival

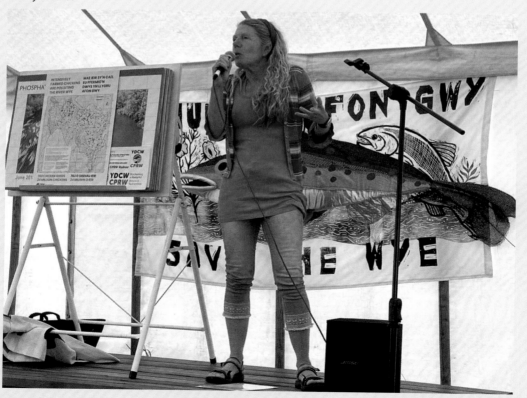

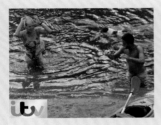
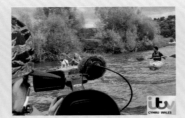
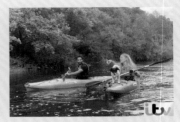

ITV Coast & Country, so much fun showing Sean Fletcher the delights of the Wye Kayaking and Wild Swimming.

Media, Me and Jack

"During our many years and adventures together, Jack and I have – to our amusement – attracted a lot of interest from the media".

We have always been happy to share the wonders of our wild adventurous life with everyone as it enables us to continue to promote the importance of connecting gently with, and respecting our fragile environment. Our relationship with Nature is one we cherish and nurture constantly.

We have worked with many celebrities on a wide variety of TV and radio programmes, have written numerous articles and had more interviews than I can recall, as interest in our wild lifestyle grew.

I have never been interested in using this attention to grow my business but instead to raise awareness of the necessity to protect the environment that makes 'the great outdoors' so special – for all of us.

Nature is kind enough to let not only Jack and I play in her gigantic garden, but everyone who wants to. When she provides so many health benefits and nurtures us so selflessly, it's only right that we reciprocate. And I'm so grateful for all the unexpected opportunities the media has given me to spread this message to the furthest and wildest corners.

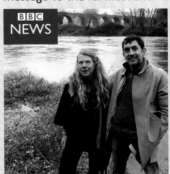

BBC News with climate editor Justin Rowlatt.

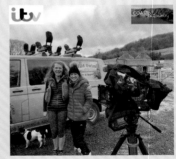

ITV Coast & Country Ruth Wignall embraces Winter swimming and Kayaking

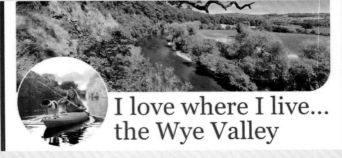

I love where I live... the Wye Valley

Magazine article

TWO Border Lives

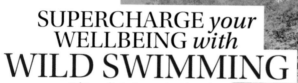

BBC 2 Border Lives part of a 5-part series following Jack and I in work and play

SUPERCHARGE *your* WELLBEING *with* WILD SWIMMING

Taking a dip in the great outdoors has amazing benefits for both body and mind, says Angela Jones

Who hasn't rolled up their trouser legs to take a quick paddle in the sea? But for many of us, the idea of submerging ourselves in a cold lake is a little out of our comfort zone. However, according to wild swim specialist, Angela Jones (swimwildwye.co.uk) it's one of the best things we can do for our wellbeing. "Taking ourselves away from modern life and back to basics in the great outdoors is second to none mentally and physically," she says.

"Wild swimming is great for circulation and boosting your metabolism, as well as strengthening your immune system. It acts as a natural anti-inflammatory and gives you a fantastic natural high. It's even said to help with menopause symptoms."

Angela has been swimming in The River Wye in England and Wales for more than 30 years and taking groups on wild swimming adventures for nearly a decade. "There is a non-competitive element to my sessions," she says. "To have fun and enjoy the wild side is paramount, if we stand and stare, everything is right in front of us."

"Nature has a way of putting its arms around us but it has a big stony toe to show us who's boss, too"

And the good news is, when it comes to wild swimming age is no barrier. Angela herself is 54 and she works with all ages and abilities. "I believe strengthening and technique can be introduced at any age and benefits the whole body whatever we do," she adds.

Tempted? There are few things you need to know before you get started. "Wild swimming is not the same as pool swimming," Angela warns. "It can be incredibly dangerous to just head into an unknown body of water. Extreme low temperatures, not being able to touch the sides, underwater currents and obstacles, and rapidly changing weather conditions are all factors that can put you at risk."

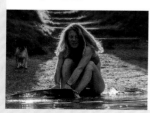

Natural Health Magazine. A great magazine to share my wild well being swim adventure knowledge.

Here are a few little media clips of some fun times filming.

Garmin Ant Middleton - I was asked to be SAS hardman Ant's Wild swim and Kayak specialist for 3 days shooting the new Garmin watch.

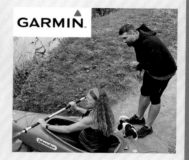

Kate Humble: Green Life, Good Life, Channel 5; always a pleasure to work with Kate!

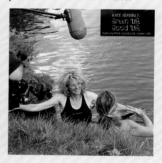

BBC Weatherman Walking with Derek Brockway: what a beautiful person - this was an absolute BLAST !!!

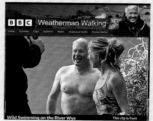

At Seas, Streams, Rivers and Lakes: Play Safe!!

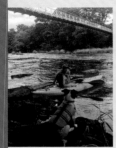

Have lots of fun and also take lots of care. Play safe!

There is nothing better than sharing your outdoor adventures with your four-legged friend but you'll have more peace of mind during "wild swimming" and boating activities if your dog's wearing a properly fitted, good-quality canine life jacket.

Be vigilant. Having fun can be exhausting — other points to remember include:

• Keep your dog out of water that you wouldn't swim in yourself. Beware of toxic algae blooms, submerged, hidden dangerous objects (on which a dog could be impaled or cut) and areas that are guarded by aggressive wildlife.

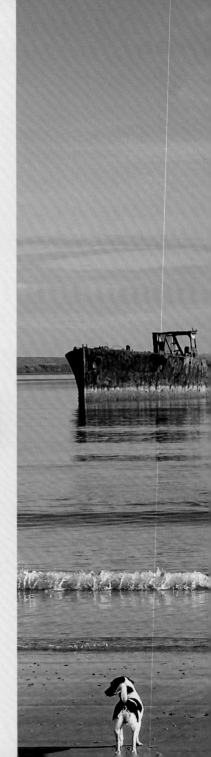

• Don't allow your dog to harass water fowl or any local wildlife.

• Continually monitor your dog In the rivers and oceans, where hazards can be more numerous and swimming can be more tiring, so watch for signs of fatigue, including trembling, heavy panting and/or swimming lower in the water or slower than usual.

• Don't encourage your dog to venture far from river's edge or offshore. That means, don't throw retriever toys and floats way out into the water. In the sea and rivers, your dog is vulnerable to rough currents, waves, riptides and cross-currents, any of which can be deadly.

• If your dog is a toy breed or has short legs or a short muzzle, it is always advisable to put them into a life jacket, whether or not they intend to go into the water — just in case.

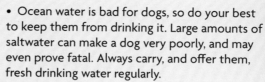
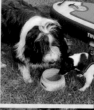

• Ocean water is bad for dogs, so do your best to keep them from drinking it. Large amounts of saltwater can make a dog very poorly, and may even prove fatal. Always carry, and offer them, fresh drinking water regularly.

• Likewise, while your dog may love rolling in stinky fish and other disgusting things that wash up on the beach or river edge, never let them eat anything. Dead fish and other marine life can contain deadly toxins.

• Be aware of the strength of the sun. Over-exposure can be as hazardous to dogs as it is to humans. Seek shade throughout the day and apply a canine-specific sun-block to vulnerable dogs 30 minutes before going in the sun, and reapply as necessary. But please check it is not harmful to aquatics – we need to be respectful of and care for ALL life.

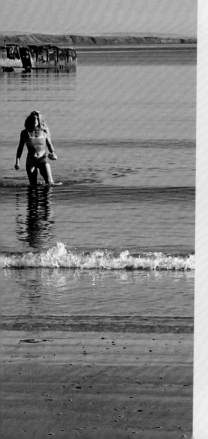

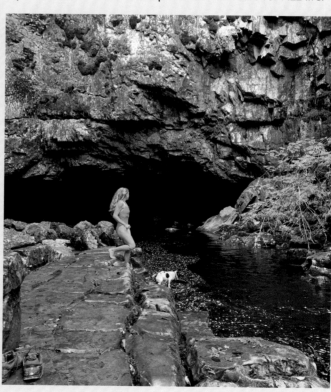

Monofins...

"SO MANY PEOPLE ARE UNAWARE OF THE WONDERS AND WILDLIFE THAT LIES BENEATH THE SURFACE"

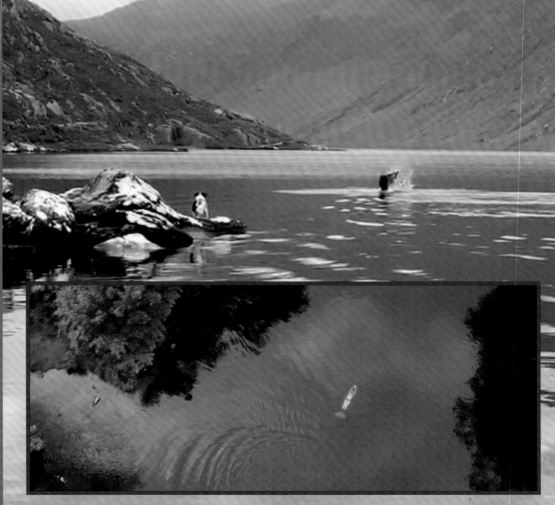

Glenbeg Lake, Ardgroom, on the Beara peninsula

Free diving fun with my four-legged friend:

As well as fully embracing all aspects of 'wild waters', the solitude and freedom of what lies beneath the surface has always been a deep passion of mine.

To enable me to explore this underworld to the best of my ability, my Monofins have played a big roll in my and Jack's life. As I enjoy the freedom of exploring below the surface of the water, my little adventurous pal Jack cheerfully swims above me, waiting for me to surface to draw a new breath and always being so pleased to see me.

I have been watching and monitoring the life below the water surface for decades. So many people are unaware of the wonders and wildlife that lies beneath the surface. We are fortunate to host some of the most beautiful deep pools and underwater rock formations, all teeming with, fascinating aquatic life. My Monofins allow me to access it all with ease and all whilst my beautiful, four-legged friend Jack, enjoys swimming on the surface above me.

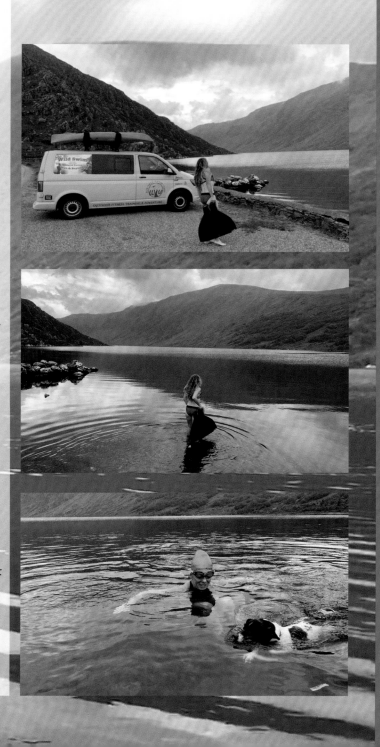

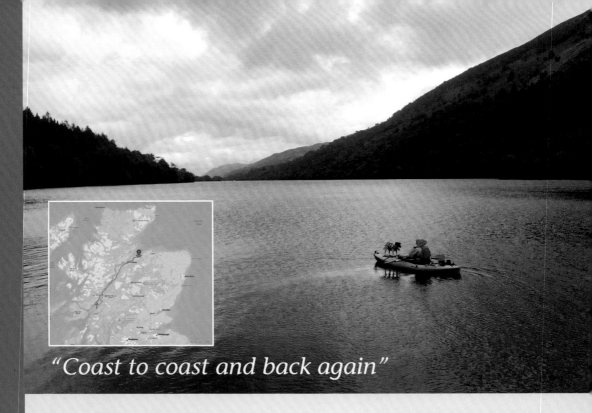

"Coast to coast and back again"

Angela and Jack's Adventures in Scotland

Every now and then we pack up, no planning, no time scale, just off we go; normally for around 5 weeks at a time.

I've always loved playing in Scotland and so love the freedom to roam with rugged ragidness and the most amazing wildlife.

So this trip I had decided to head to Scotland for our next adventure. I had been there many times before, swimming and kayaking the lochs, rivers and coastlines, and bouncing around some wonderful mountains with my Jack in tow. We had totally enjoyed the freedom of kipping out in our bivvy bag and being at one with the most wonderful encounters with wildlife.

I had an idea about crossing Scotland this time, I wanted to

join the Atlantic to the North Sea with my kayak so I had to think of rough logistics. I don't map read because I never want to become regimental or put too much emphasis on times, locations and goals, and also being dyslexic it's pretty much impossible. I'm very much about the here and now and the enjoyment that it holds!

I knew I had a parachute harness in my garage; I knew I had a set of wheels for my kayak; and I knew that if I some how connected my harness to my kayak and attached it to wheels I could tow it. So for a couple of weeks I devised

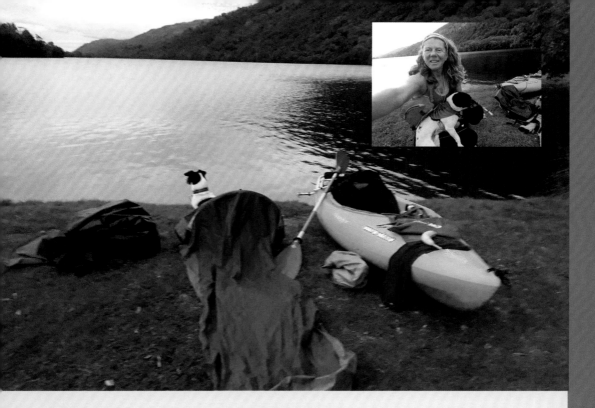

a very bodged set-up to do just that. Jack was always such a chilled dog he would always look at me and I could tell it was "What's she up to now?" After our long days on the river taking clients wild swimming and kayaking we would always be up to our own fun play time too.

We would run around our sleepy village where we lived, kayak on tow, and the Wild Woman of the Wye and her little pooch would be just who they were – rather eccentric and a little bit crazy. My thoughts for lumpy mountain sections, returning with kayak across Scottish mountains would be to carry the kayak on my back with harness, if I couldn't tow with wheels. So we replicated this back at home on a few test runs!

When August 4th came we headed to Scotland and I had to think about Coast to Coast "Atlantic to North Sea". I loaded our VW van up with everything we might need and off we set, two days later arriving off the coast of Scotland, where I found a good place to get my head down and launch our adventure early next morning at the mouth of Loch Linnhe. I didn't want to do just the Caledonian Canal – I wanted to join up the Atlantic and North Sea, and Loch Linnhe and the Moray Firth allowed me to do just this: and obviously make it adaptable to my little Jack's capability.

The weather was rough and there were a couple of big storms in August. The west to east crossing was ten days of battling the elements, with wind gusts of up to 80 miles an hour. Not only did we hit rough waters but the backwash from the large cruise boats threw us around, being hit by waves in all directions .

We tucked in along the shore for our night's camp and one particular night we were pretty trashed after fighting the elements all day.

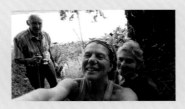

That evening as we were ready to get into our bivvy bag, rather tired, a beautiful elderly couple appeared from nowhere and asked us what on earth we were up to? They said it was their land and pointed to a small light on the side of the hill which they lived behind. They were so warm and friendly and invited us in for a cuppa and cake, which was the best cake we had tasted as we were living on very bland food from our kayak store. The next day they came down to see us off and wished us luck on our way; we will never forget their warmth.

We battled on and rode the weather and the waves, vigilant at all times for those big old boats with monstrous motors. We travelled through the Caledonia Canal, with Jack as Captain as usual, and then retreating below splash deck in choppy waters.

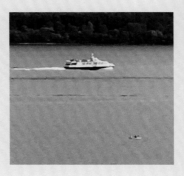

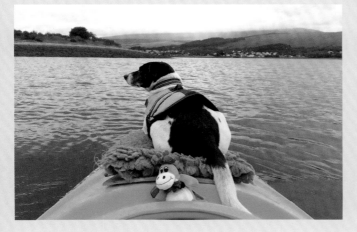

We managed eventually to get all the way to the last sea lock: it was howling with wind and rain and our reward was a golden key from the Lock Master who had been told we were coming through. I still use the key to this day: it opens up every canal washroom in the country!!

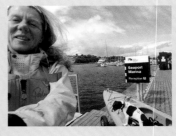

Over 100 miles of kayaking and experiencing Nature's force, with some of the wettest wild camps I've experienced, we hit Inverness. We didn't want to do just the Great Glen Way; we wanted to really explore west to east!! We had the best time ever, with great evening and early morning swims to bookend our days!

We shared our wild camps with the sight of remarkable wildlife and serenity that is hard to describe. Jack and I ate on and off the kayak and played at every minute.

Eventually, reaching Nairn we came out and realised the Highland Games were in progress! What a treat, first time for us both and tossing the caber was a must to watch. The strapping kilted winner took a liking to my Jack and gave him a bit of a Scottish cuddle: Jack was not amused! After a short day on the beach

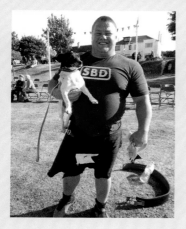

camping and chilling, we knew we had to head over those little lumpy mountains back to base!!

It was fairly exhilarating to turn round and start running back, kayak in tow! I clipped the parachute straps on, winched it to the kayak, added wheels and off we set.
My plan was to allow my woof

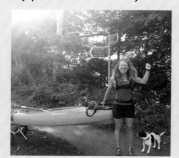

to get rest in the kayak when it was being towed on wheels. "Was it heck", Jack was so not having any of that; he wanted to walk and run by my side. It's perfect when you have no time restriction or mission; like all our adventures, we did it at our own pace and always made it fun! Being so in tune with my Jack he would always let me know what he wanted – rest, play, food – we were very in tune with each other's thoughts.

As long as I was back within 5 weeks and we were safe, nothing else came into the equation.

We Joined up with the Great Glen Way and kept going down from Fort William to Loch Linnhe and Oban where our base of our VW van was.

It's very much like life – it's great fun and you don't know what you're going to come up against as you've never done it before! The unknown is intriguing and my favourite phrase is "even when you're falling, you're going forward." Strong body, strong head.

The whole journey was totally amazing and challenging. It pushed me to the limits at times but it was always good fun, including sleeping out under the stars in my bivvy bag... in plenty of rain.

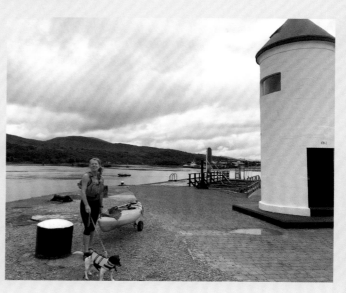

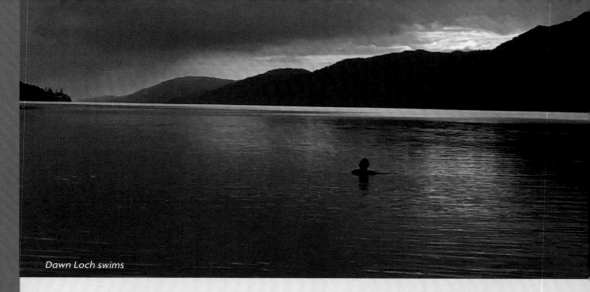

Dawn Loch swims

My daily morning and night loch swims were totally magical. And the Scots were truly welcoming... they thought I was pretty crazy for the adventure that I was on with my doggy!

It is so strange to be in the remotest of places and a random stranger would appear, and I was often quizzed about what we were doing.

People often ask me why I do what I do. I always think that if you're asking that question then you will never understand the answer. I also get asked, "Aren't you scared being a woman at your age and on your own?" That never comes into it and I'm not on my own, I'm with my bestie. I think scared is being in a city full of people, rushing about with no-one doing what they <u>want </u>to do, just doing what they <u>have</u> to do! My balance is very much contentment and you cannot put a price on that.

Jack's a remarkable dog – and he has had a lifetime of adventure, coming to work with me every day and going out with my clients... kayaking, wild swimming, trail running, wild camping... On this trip he was truly amazing, sitting on the front of my kayak, and under the spray deck in the really rough weather!

It was a busman's holiday for both of us! But oh so much fun.

With the huge increase in dog ownership, comes a huge increase on the affect on wildlife deterioration, with dogs allowed to run wild out of control and chase everything.

I've witnessed nesting birds be ripped apart, owners thinking it's intuitive to allow water fowl to be chased and killed. I taught Jack to respect and protect wildlife, but at the drop of a command he would turn on a rat if I asked.

Dogs know right from wrong and just like a child this can be taught. The increase in dog ownership through lock-down has had a very concerning affect on the great outdoors.

Not saying we are all guilty but we so need to respect our invitation into the great outdoors.

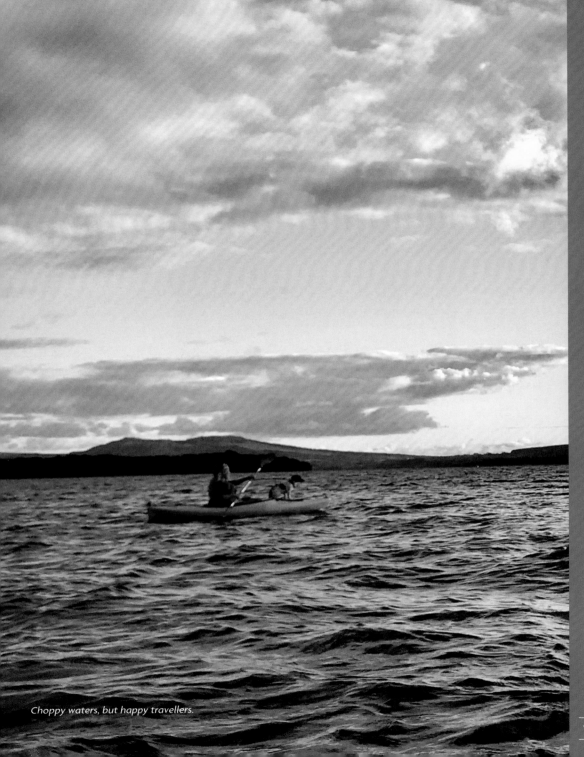

Choppy waters, but happy travellers.

ANGELA JONES

The term 'busman's holiday' is frequently heard in the world of paddlesports – where the only difference between 'work' and 'holiday' is the presence of clients, and even then there's sometimes some crossover! However, Angela Jones has taken the term to a whole new level. She runs www.Run-Wild.co.uk on the Wye, offering coaching in outdoor fitness, running, wild swimming and kayaking throughout the year. So you'd think if she had a 5-week summer break she might head off for a relaxing holiday. Nope, she spent 32 days exploring the Wye; kayaking 100 miles down, running 160 miles back from Chepstow to the Cambrian Mountains, then swimming 84 miles down. Wild camping along the way. This year was a similar 'holiday', just a little further north. Kayaking the Scottish coast-to-coast, from Loch Linnhe into the Caledonian Canal and then to the Moray Firth. This route is a classic canoe trip but Angela wanted to join the Atlantic to the North Sea by starting at Loch Linnhe, a tidal loch. And, rather than arranging a shuttle (like most boaters), when she finished the paddle she strapped a pair of wheels onto her kayak, turned round and jogged her way back along 92 miles of the Great Glen Way. All her adventures over the last 8 years have been shared with her faithful little Jack Russell terrier, Jack, who can always be found in his favourite position perched on front of her kayak. Ceufad managed to get her away from the water to find out a bit more about this remarkably modest and inspirational serial doorstep adventurer.

It sounds like you love the outdoors – where did the interest come from?

I've always loved the outdoors and the freedom it brings, particularly the wildlife and the spontaneous adventures. I could never understand why I couldn't be out there all day everyday, and would often gaze out of classroom windows and yearn for the freedom to explore. I remember when I was 14 a careers officer asking what I wanted to be. I replied that I wanted to explore and travel, and she just laughed and said that won't pay the bills!

At the age of 30 after travelling on and off for years around Africa and Asia, and working in Middle East taking adventure holidays for a company, I returned to UK. My personality is very spur-of-the-moment and constantly loves engaging in new adventures. I had been swimming for years, so I took up running and then triathlon. This very quickly took me from 14 stone to an international athlete travelling to many countries. Before the age of 30 I had never run and definitely hadn't heard of triathlon!

So it's not just about exploration and adventure – you compete as well?

I've been competing nationally and internationally for over 20 years in many disciplines including running, mountain, trail, road, cross country, track, triathlon, duathlon, aquathon, swimming and cycling.
In my first few years of running I was selected for my country and also for triathlon. I never take competing too seriously as it's all about the pleasure for me, and that goes for everything I do.

That's quite a competitive career. What are your highlights and biggest achievements?

One highlight has to be turning up at a race unaware it was a selection event for the Worlds at senior level in mountain running. And at the end being asked could I travel to Alaska and run for my country. Another would be my first triathlon – borrowing a bike, putting Vaseline on the chain ... basically not having a clue about anything and then beating the Welsh champion!

Over 22 years of competing every single race, be it swimming, running, cycling, duathlons triathlons or aquathons has been a highlight.
I have been known to race up to 50 times a year and they are all great fun and great experiences. I have never set training schedules. No distances, no speeds. Just what I want to do when I want to do it. Always solo.
This has changed in the last 2 years, where competition has taken a back stage and the wild calls even more.
As for achievements I race a lot and have won quite a few (*numerous – ed*) national and international titles.
I've been selected for several World Championships for my country in mountain running and triathlon. I've also competed in the 1st Commonwealth Games in mountain running. I won Gold in the Worlds GB team in my age group for mountain running at 50. And being selected for my first Wales World Mountain Running Team in Alaska. still producing some of my best times at 50!

And somehow you manage to fit kayaking in as well?
I have been river kayaking for over 20 years; it gives me the freedom to enjoy the wildlife and its surroundings. It's a totally different perspective from wild swimming but gives me time to enjoy the water in a different format. Often if I'm kayaking and find an interesting section I just slip in and free dive into salmon pools. It allows me to watch the fish and the cormorants diving.

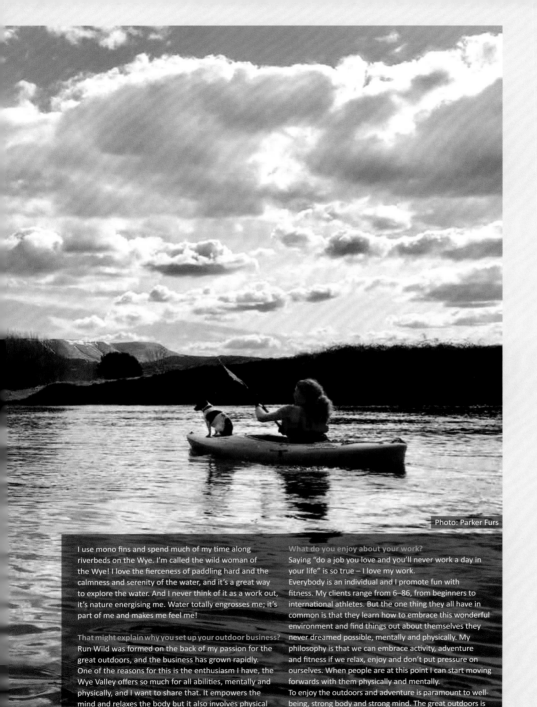

Photo: Parker Furs

I use mono fins and spend much of my time along riverbeds on the Wye. I'm called the wild woman of the Wye! I love the fierceness of paddling hard and the calmness and serenity of the water, and it's a great way to explore the water. And I never think of it as a work out, it's nature energising me. Water totally engrosses me; it's part of me and makes me feel me!

That might explain why you set up your outdoor business?
Run Wild was formed on the back of my passion for the great outdoors, and the business has grown rapidly. One of the reasons for this is the enthusiasm I have, the Wye Valley offers so much for all abilities, mentally and physically, and I want to share that. It empowers the mind and relaxes the body but it also involves physical activity. Plus no two days are the same and the seasons are so beautiful.

What do you enjoy about your work?
Saying "do a job you love and you'll never work a day in your life" is so true – I love my work.
Everybody is an individual and I promote fun with fitness. My clients range from 6–86, from beginners to international athletes. But the one thing they all have in common is that they learn how to embrace this wonderful environment and find things out about themselves they never dreamed possible, mentally and physically. My philosophy is that we can embrace activity, adventure and fitness if we relax, enjoy and don't put pressure on ourselves. When people are at this point I can start moving forwards with them physically and mentally.
To enjoy the outdoors and adventure is paramount to well-being, strong body and strong mind. The great outdoors is my office and I feel privileged to share this with others. It excites me everyday to share my playground with others.

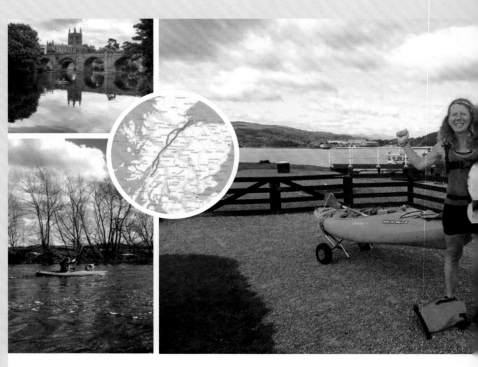

Sounds fantastic! What's your typical working day?

Everyday I river swim with clients, I kayak and do outdoor fitness on the banks of the Wye. I work 6 days a week averaging 7 to 10 hours a daily of activities with clients, as well as wild camps. I do exactly the same when I am not with clients, so I really don't class any of it as work!

It seems like the Wye is a very special place to you?

The Wye runs through my veins. I swim in it every day. I sleep on its banks or in its woods most weeks. I kayak it and run it. The rock formations and wildlife are second to none. It's the one true place I feel totally at one with.

That might explain your Wye adventure last year – how did that come about?

Every year I take August off, and the year before I was doing a pretty similar trip around the Outer Hebrides. The year before that was the Inner Hebrides and north Scotland. I have the personality of being very spontaneous and chilled, and I'm also dyslexic, which helps with not over-analysing, so I never plan. Literally a couple days before my 2017 August break I just thought I'd play on my favourite river for 5 weeks! I thought I love kayaking it,

so I'll kayak it. Then I thought but I also love swimming it … and running it … and also wild camping. In the end I thought right, let's just go up and down doing all 3, and sleep out. So I hid a bit of kit in the woods in two sections and carried the rest in my kayak. I slept in a bivvy bag so travelled light and lived pretty much on tinned tuna and rice pudding. I set no time scale, distance or plans. All I knew was that I had 5 weeks till my next clients, so had a long play ahead.

> Life excites me and everday I feel blessed that at 52 I have more energy and zest than I've ever had.

It sounds like your Scotland trip this summer had a similar start?

That was a spontaneous trip as well! I knew I wanted to join up the west of Scotland with the east by water. From the Atlantic to the North Sea. And then get back to start point by carrying my kayak on my back.

And what happened?

A four-week solo adventure in August with my loyal companion Jack. Starting at Loch Linnhe, then through to the Caledonian Canal and into the Moray Firth, which goes into

the North Sea. I didn't want to do just the Caledonian Canal – I wanted to join up the Atlantic and North Sea, and Loch Linnhe and the Moray Firth allowed me to do this.

And Jack joined you on this adventure too?

Yes! He's a remarkable dog – at 9 years old he has had a lifetime of adventure, coming to work with me everyday and going out with my clients … kayaking, wild swimming, trail running, wild camping … On this trip he was truly amazing, sitting on the front of my kayak, and under the spray deck in the really rough weather! It was a busman's holiday for both of us!

Rough weather – weren't there a couple of storms in August?

The west to east crossing was 10 days of battling the elements, with wind gusts of up to 80 miles an hour.

After that it must have been fairly tough to turn round and start running back, whilst towing your kayak?

No, not really. It's very much like life – it's great fun and you don't know what you're going to come up against as you've never done it before! The unknown is intriguing and my favourite phrase is "even when

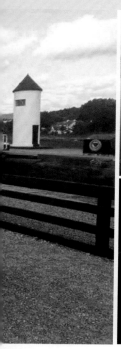
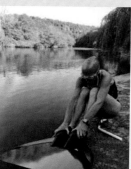
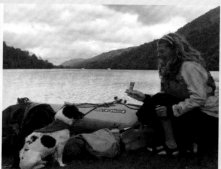
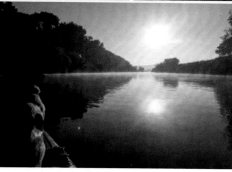
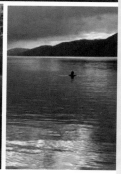

you're falling, you're going forward." Strong body, strong head.

Was it worth it?

The whole journey was totally amazing and challenging. It pushed me to the limits at times but it was always good fun, including sleeping out under the stars in my bivvy bag ... in plenty of rain. My daily morning and night loch swims were totally magical. And the Scots were truly welcoming ... and thought I was pretty crazy for the adventure that I was on.

Do you get quizzed about what you're doing?

People often ask me why I do what I do. I always think that if you're asking that question then you will never understand the answer. I also get asked "aren't you scared being a woman at your age and on your own?" That never comes into it. I think scared is being in a city full of people, rushing about with no-one doing what they want to do, just doing what they have to do!

I work with everyone and anyone, from well-known actors and comedians, to many well-to-do clients, and also the average wonderful person. My balance is very much contentment and you cannot put a price on that.

Your trips sound fantastic – do you share them with your clients?

Yes, but wild-camping is optional! I run adventure experiences on the Wye and in Castellar de la Frontera in southern Spain. Clients can choose their activities and trip duration, so they are completely tailor-made.

> I'm a solo adventurer with Jack the Dog. Contentment is when you feel totally at peace and most people associate this with partners but for some it's finding yourself in mind and body.

The Spanish trip is really special – it's in a 12th century hill-top castle that's been converted into a hotel. It's in a nature reserve too so the wildlife and scenery are amazing. We usually finish the trip with a night at the coast, staying on a yacht and enjoying the dolphins. But if clients want to wild-camp on the Wye then I can arrange that too!

So ... any plans for next year?

I've just spent 8 days in Iceland ice swimming and sleeping out with the fantastic wildlife. I managed the most amazing swims in 2C

water. Including swimming between the two tectonic plates, which has never been done before in a swimming costume (to my knowledge!). I also free dived with mono fins. And swam in the North Atlantic and icefalls! I will be taking 3 weeks off at Christmas and always wait till the last minute to see what interesting places I can fly to. Last Christmas I flew out to Caribbean and visited 11 islands; free diving, kayaking, running and exploring these beautiful places.

This is the third chapter in my life and it's an amazing journey of the most interesting things. Life is for living and we should never be scared to explore. However, the Wye is my home and I have the same passion for it as the first time I set eyes on it 32 years ago!

ANGELA JONES

www.angelajonesswimwild.co.uk

My early years and international Jack

From the age of 32, and for over twenty years, I unintentionally became an International athlete. I raced several times at Senior World Level, doing a bit of each discipline, including, mountain running, cross country triathlon, swimming, duathlon, aquathon and cycling.

Coaches and fellow athletes would often say, "If you concentrated on one thing, you'd be unstoppable." But maybe I didn't want to be.

Nature is my home, my training ground and my playground and it definitely enhances my soul, so to be able to share that with my 'woof' for 15 years was a true pleasure – and my 'gold medal'.

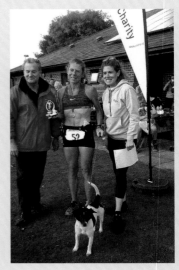

As a child, I remember looking at my Labrador and thinking we are very much dictated to and governed by everything we 'have to do' or are 'expected to do' in our lives, and wouldn't it be so much nicer not to be 'owned' or have a set routine, and instead to have the freedom to go on many fun adventures together?

When I was 13, a careers teacher asked me what I wanted to do when I left school and I remember saying "to live a life of adventure." She replied, "That won't pay the bills." "What a load of cobblers", I thought.

For eleven years, I detested school and couldn't understand what I had done wrong to be in such an awful place. My comfort was my Golden Labrador, Cindy. When I came home, she was big and soft and comforting – and knew what I was thinking. We would have the most wonderful walks, where I would do plenty of gazing and dreaming.

I've lived on my own since 15 years of age; from 16, I was pinging around the world solo, randomly travelling the Middle East, Africa, Asia and anywhere else my curious mind and trusty rucksack took me. Accepting and adapting to my challenging surroundings toughened me up and taught me to appreciate every wonderful moment. This was 'proper education'.
Often on my travels I would see dogs of all breeds, shapes and sizes and many that were suffering from malnutrition. I would often spend time feeding them, and talking to them as I pulled the ticks from their matted coats – it always played on my heart.

I continued to bob around the world, discovering, seeking, and curiously embracing countries and cultures. But all through my travels and many different episodes in life, it was a wild life. Nature adventures always enthused and engulfed me with a feeling of belonging. I don't know why or how it had that effect and I've never over-analysed it, it just did.

After so much travelling, my love for my homeland drew me back like a magnet and I knew it was a place like no other in the world.

As I've played all over the world, swimming in different locations, from sub-zero temperatures at the tectonic plates in Iceland to crossing the Wild Atlantic Way in Ireland, my heart has always belonged to Mother Nature. I taste her sweetness; I feel her strengths, her moods, her solitude, her pain. The changing seasons, the increase in tourists, the migration of the birds – I watch it all from above, and below the water.

My philosophy, which runs through my life, is to never take yourself too seriously – great things are achieved when you relax. A smile and enjoyment run through everything I do like rivers run through the valleys. I have always had the imagination and sense of adventure to make things fun and relaxed, and that's when the everyday things develop into a habit.

My four-legged friend, Jack was a part of my international and adventurous life for 15 years and we shared the most amazing journey together.

I feel very protective of our beautiful countryside and landscapes. I wrote this book to introduce others to the beauty and joys of sharing wild adventures – and which are even better when shared with your best friend or your 'woof'. In this book – as in my life outside the pages – I offer advice on enjoying wild swimming, kayaking, paddle boarding, wild camping and trails and most importantly, whilst always respecting the environment and caring for your dog.

The well-documented health benefits of the great outdoors are vast and to be able to share these with your bestie, your 'woof', is a very special gift and will build the most beautiful bond between you.

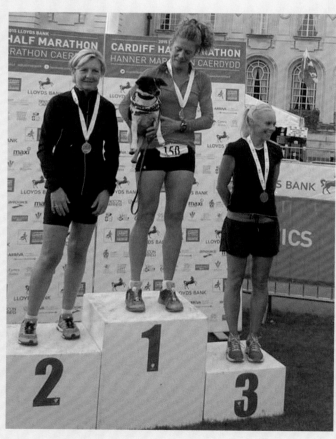

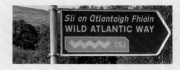

Angela and Jack's Adventures in Ireland

I had never spent much time in Ireland but knew it was a place that I wanted to explore with Jack – and in a way that allowed us the time to give it the respect it deserved.

So one of our '5 week blocks' that I set aside for exploring, had to be invested in heading out to the southern shores of the Emerald Isle. Once again we opted for 'no planning'; just left home for Fishguard, for the crossing to Rosslaire. Our VW van was full of all the essential adventure kit that Jack and I would need, along with plenty of energy and enthusiasm for our 5-week window of wandering and exploration.

We always have this wonderful feeling of not knowing what's ahead, and the gift of knowing that we just have this quality, magical, unrushed time together. Of course, the beauty of being self contained in our trusty VW van meant that we could stop anywhere we liked and had all the equipment on board to adapt to any adventurous situation that took our fancy! Whether it was swimming, kayaking, wild camping, hiking, or even enjoying my mono fins, there was nothing we couldn't do – whenever we wanted to do it.

The only way to explain my and Jack's life together is to say that we've always felt and shared the excitement and thrill of being free whilst being totally connected to each other and the adventures of life.

By chance we slipped onto The Wild Atlantic Way and loved what we discovered. The people were friendly and the scenery was spectacular – and so we soon settled cheerfully and comfortably into our familiar nomadic ways.

We kayaked a lot, which enabled us to reach small remote islands and all their wonderful wildlife along the way. Around every corner we stumbled across lakes with their crystal clear waters and one of our favourite things was to start the day by slipping quietly out of our cosy, warm sleeping bag straight into the clear, cool water.

Kayaking out to Ballycotton Island

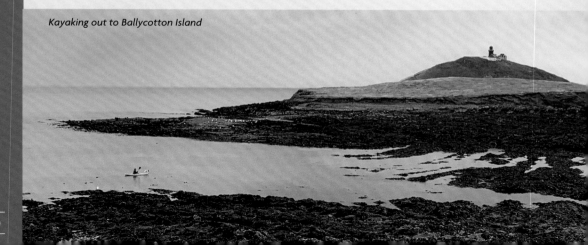

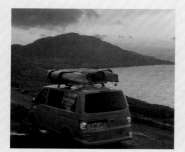

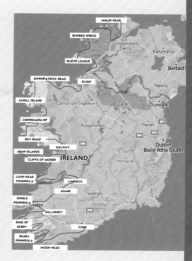

We certainly enjoyed some 'extreme exploring' and saw the most magical sights, including Ballycotton which was also a great favourite of ours. We kayaked out to the island and respectfully enjoyed its beautiful clear waters and its wildlife. We were rewarded with the most beautiful full moon swim and were entertained by Oyster-Catchers. The Atlantic views from our bivvy bag in the mornings were just glorious; but after 3 days we knew we had to move on as there was so much more to see and experience: star-light kayaking in the bioluminescent waters of Lough Hyne in Co. Cork, which was pretty spectacular.

We had herring throwing themselves at us as they were attracted to the light from my head torch and they landed with a 'thlop' on our kayak. True to character, Jack was totally unphased and respected their brief visits. We spent 5 glorious days in this area enjoying Ireland's first Nature Reserve, with plenty of early morning swims and bioluminescent night swims in the 50m deep salt water. Water which connects to the sea and therefore fills up twice a day and then drains down a narrow gorge. Nature provided some exciting kayaking, and the sheltered reefs added much excitement to some free diving with my mono fins allowing me to go deeper. All the time Jack would swim on the surface waiting for me to bob back up. The trails from here are pretty spectacular and Knockomagh Hill provided a stunning place to enjoy a peaceful couple of nights in our bivvy bag, watching the sun set on Lough Hyne.

We were totally enthralled by the whole Beara Peninsula, which is a truly stunning coastal route with mind-blowing, breathtaking views, rugged wild mountains – which we hiked and ran together – and mystical heritage sites like the Ardgroom Stone Circle.

Dursey Island was another beautiful island and where Jack and I went over to it via an old, cranky pull lift and we managed to get a glimpse of our first whale of the trip off the West of the island.

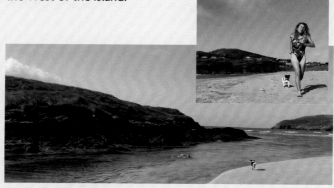

Angela swimming down the Estuary into the sea, while Jack runs and joins her.

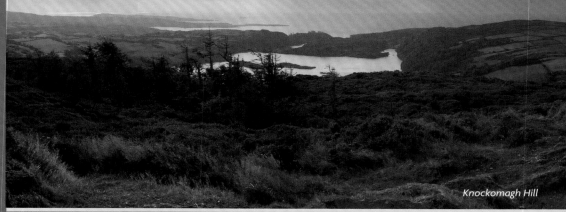

Knockomagh Hill

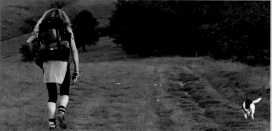

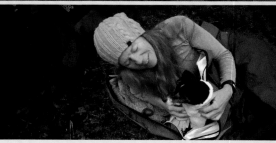

We spent much of our 5-week adventure bobbing in and around the coast, and during one early morning swim at Garnish beach we gently ventured into a small harbour. As we bobbed up in the water next to a boat unloading its fresh morning catch, the local fisherman kindly asked if we would like a fresh fish for our breakfasts. I felt a bit like a seal, but gratefully accepted, and Jack and I shared a very tasty breakfast that morning.

Water water everywhere! Farranamanagh Lough Kilcrohane next to Dunmanus Bay was a magical double-swim fun day with plenty of exciting wildlife to indulge our heart and eyes.

There are so many memories to cherish; like meandering and swimming down the estuary together to the sea at Barley Cove. It was pretty special and we enjoyed a shared lunch of beans and tuna straight from the cans, on the beach. It may sound 'yuk' to some people but it's the sort of 'fine dining' that we've always done together and enjoyed hugely.

During one of our hikes we came across a rather strange farmer on a remote hill farm who wanted a kiss – yuk!

Jack soon showed him that although he may be a little dog, he had a big ferocious bark!

Every time we got a little too close to towns, we always headed back out to quiet land. We learned the wonderful way of the Irish and always greeted them in the same way they welcomed Jack and I – with a hearty "Good Morning to ya!"

My VW van is sign written with "Wild Swim Specialist' and I remember an elderly man with a puzzled face asking, "Why would anyone pay you to go swimming? We do it over here for free all the time."

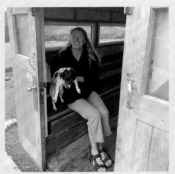

Dursey Island, Cable Car

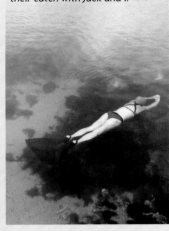

Early morning swim in Garnish bay where the fishermen shared their catch with Jack and I.

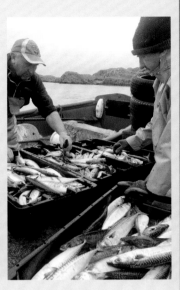

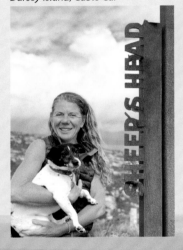

It made me chuckle as it was true - everyone in Ireland embraced the water like cleaning their teeth – it was something that came so naturally to them.

Ireland was a total joy for us both, where we made more of the most magical memories and we came away knowing that one day we would return.

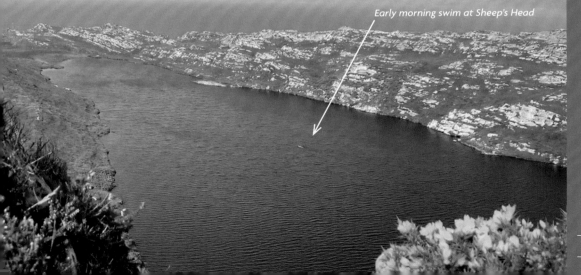

Early morning swim at Sheep's Head

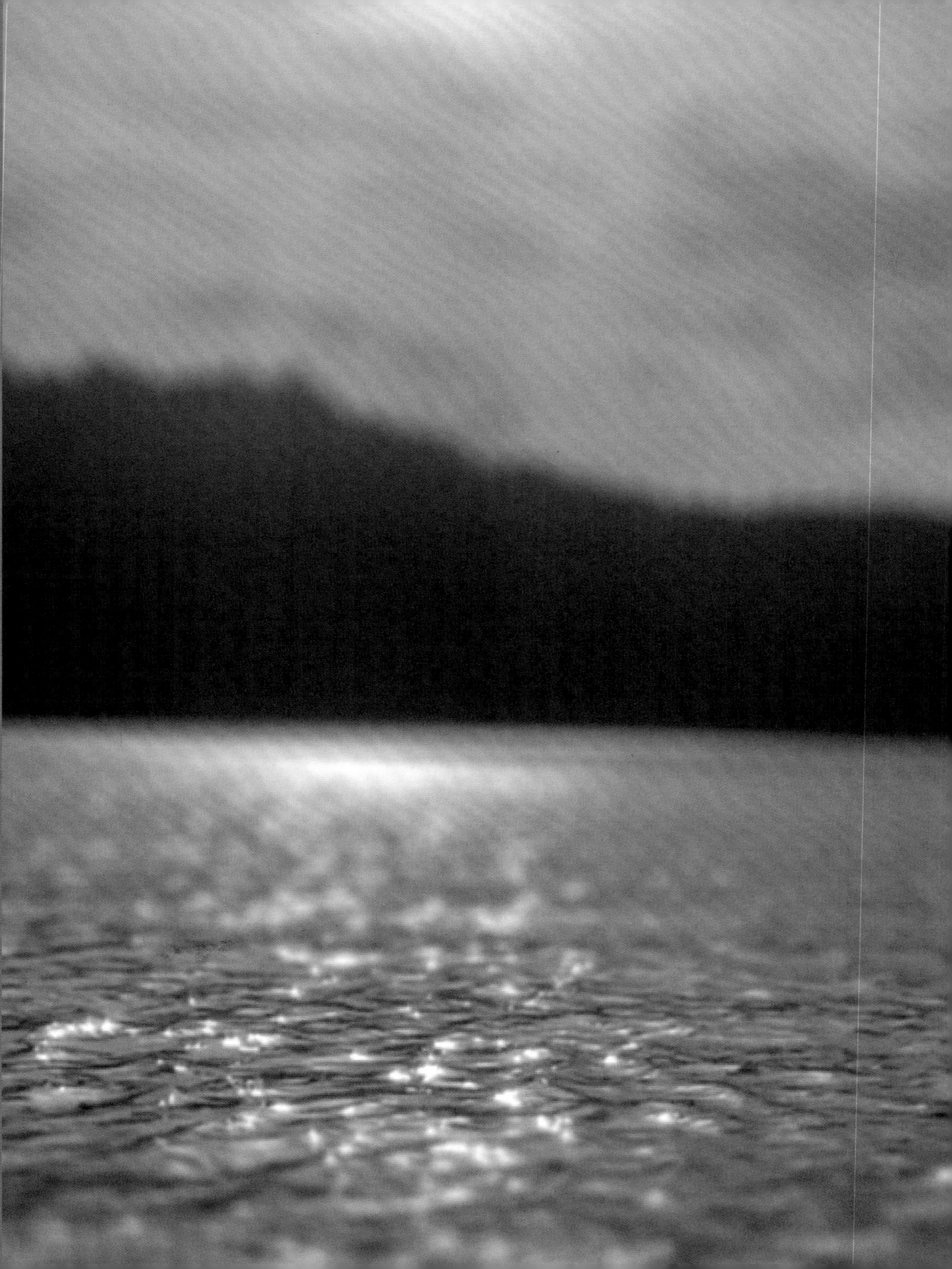

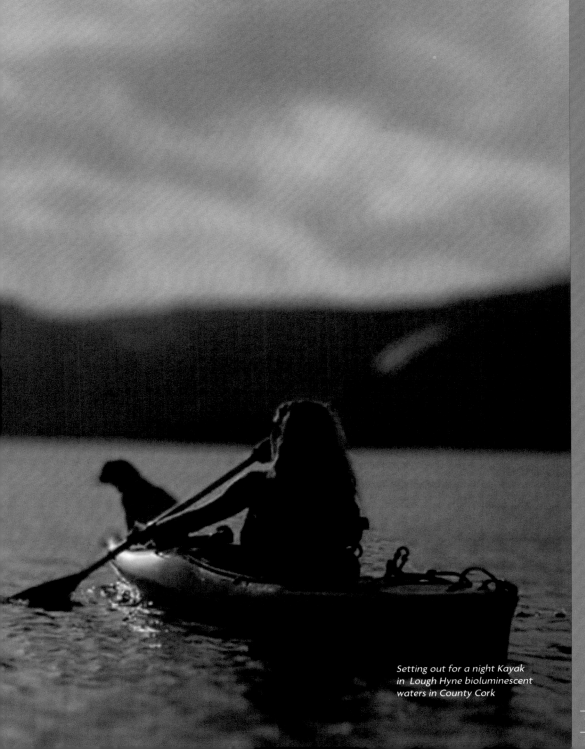

Setting out for a night Kayak in Lough Hyne bioluminescent waters in County Cork

Five wonderful weeks spent exploring my favourite river, 'The Wye.'

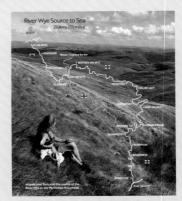

This adventure exploring the wonderful Wye was, in many ways, another Busman's Holiday where I spontaneously 'shut up shop' one day, hid some 'adventure kit' in carefully placed barrels along 3 sections of the 155 miles of the River Wye before toddling off to play on a 5-week adventure with Jack. My favourite saying is, "I never get lost as I never know where I'm going," but the beauty of this adventure was that I know the river like the back of my hand. For over four decades it's been a huge part of my life and I so, so wanted to invest time to indulge and even overdose on its pure magical beauty. So, with our trusty VW van kitted up, Jack and I set off for the Cambrian Mountains and the start of another adventure. After spending our first night in the VW in the hills, we headed of on a 18-mile fun run, jogging up, down and around the magnificent Cambrian Mountains until we arrived at the source of the Wye. Our hearts nearly burst with Joy to see and drink the fresh clear water at the birthplace of our Magical River.

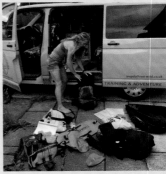

We spent the day playing in the freshly emerging Wye as it set out on its course through the mountains. The very next day we set off with our kayak, and from the stunning upper Wye, we travelled for over 100 miles along its delicious, diverse waters. Our kayak was lightly packed with the bare minimum, and Jack enjoyed watching the wildlife from his Captain's Seat at the front of the kayak. He gazed respectfully at swans, egrets, otters, kingfishers and salmon leaping and would tell me when he needed a stretch or a break from the kayak. Being so beautifully connected, I would always know just before he let me know and would always make sure he was comfortable and happy.

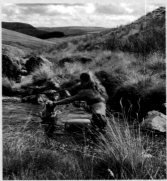

As the sun set on the Wye, and shimmered across the water, we made some wonderful wild camps – always respecting the land and its environment. We had such wonderful nights cwtched up together in our bivvy bag. We were lucky to see

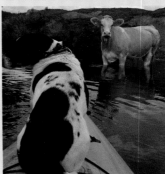

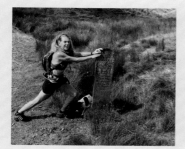

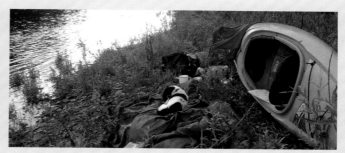

and share so much wildlife both during the day and the night and our magical swims made a nice change from kayaking.

One day, whilst kayaking down past a campsite, Jack heard children playing in the river and as he adores 'little people' we got out of the kayak to swim past them. Jack's favourite fun-trick is to dive off my back when I'm swimming, using me as a spring board – but this time as I surfaced he chose my nose as a diving board by mistake. And that resulted in a big claw-sized split across my nose and blood everywhere. It didn't bother me (or Jack) but we were filming with the BBC the next day as they made a documentary about our adventures, and I think they thought our adventures were much more dangerous than they were. Jack and I kept our secret.

Sleeping out under a bridge one rainy night, an inquisitive

fox came over to investigate but as always Jack gently alerted me to our visitor. Although on another night camp I got poked by a paddle from a curious early morning kayaker to see if I was alive in

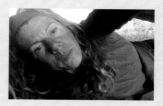

my bivvy bag, as Jack slept soundly. To this day we are still friends and still laugh about it!

Jack had spent his life on this river, for work and play and was so in-tune with the river that he could hear the change in speed and gravel rolling along the riverbed and would know when it was sensible to get below deck on the kayak! During all our adventures, Jack never barked, chased or got excited by wildlife, he would just watch, absorb, admire and enjoy – just like myself.

We spent ten days kayaking at our leisure, watching wildlife and playing with life, before eventually finishing up in Chepstow. We had a well-earned day of chilling and then set off on our 'fun run', bouncing 160 miles back to the source of the Wye. We gently passed though many untouched trails and mountain ranges, calling upon our carefully planned barrels of supplies that we had pre-hidden when necessary. We had some wonderfully feral nights out and one night whilst sleeping in a beautiful field full of tall corn with just a small tarpaulin over our heads, a little mouse paid us a visit.

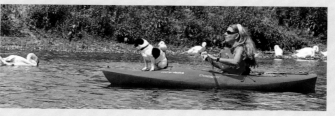

We were all perfectly happy to respect and share each other's space.

Our little adventure was so beautifully unrushed and we never had a goal or any time limits – just pure, playful fun. As we continued on our run back to source, we stopped at a lovely old converted barn to ask if we could leave some litter in their bin. We were warmly welcomed and offered tea and given home-made sloe gin in the smallest of bottles to take on our way. I didn't like to say, 'Neither Jack or I drink' and accepted it gratefully and gracefully.

As we ran through the orchards near Hereford, we shared many a scrumptious apple straight from the trees. But shhhhh! Don't tell anyone.

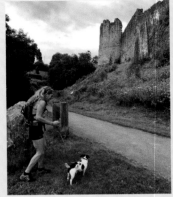

Jack and I start our run back to source from Chepstow.

We stopped running when we came to Gillfaulach Nature Reserve and took time to explore the amazing area. Above the water pools stood a solo figure and as we met and talked, this wonderful lady explained that she was a poet and recited a few poems to me and Jack. I could see why she was so inspired by this beautiful place. Full of lovely poetry, Jack and I slipped into deep, clear pools with stunning rock formations and stayed and played there for hours, just getting lost in time.

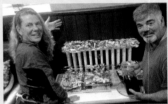

A warm welcome and sloe gin gift.

I remember one terribly wet day, taking a break from the soggy mountain running to sit down on a summit, to get a rest and gather my thoughts. Jack came over, and looked intently straight into my soul to check that I was OK. Dogs have definitely got a sixth sense and that day, he knew I was 'cooked'!

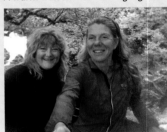

Poet we met at Gilfaulach

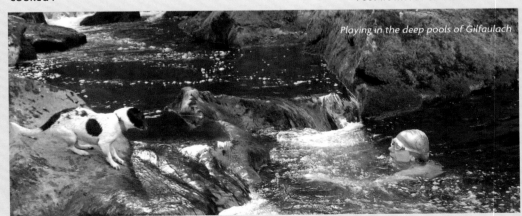

Playing in the deep pools of Gilfaulach

But Just over the very next mountain top we heard a music festival going on and that joyful, uplifting sound echoing through the valley was just what we needed. My and Jack's favourite thing has always been early morning swims where we slip straight from the warmth of our bivvy

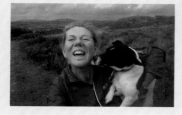

bag into the cool, refreshing river – it's just 'playful Heaven'. We stopped off at Hay Castle to meet the BBC who were following our journey and I bought Jack a bone from the butcher as a 'treat'. But Jack said, 'Yuk, no thanks' – he had never had a bone in his 10 years and wasn't going to start now.

We eventually got back to the source of our wonderful

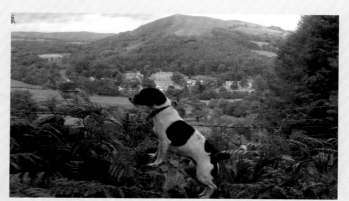

Wye and picked up our VW for a good night's sleep and quick re-charge before heading back down to swim the deeper sections of the Wye. Jack joined me for some of the shorter sections – and all of the play time - but I needed a friend to bring Jack in a kayak to catch me up along the way, as no way would I want Jack ever doing too greater distances. Your woof best friend's limits are totally different to yours and are always my priority.

As I swam downstream from Hay I remember getting slapped in the face by a salmon as I dived down into the deep pools where the Welsh and English border crosses, just below Hay town. I don't know who was the more surprised, but as always we simply respected each other and swam on.

Ten days later I had notched up over 86 miles of swimming – swirling and ottering in the mystical, meandering river. Jack and I even popped over to take part in the World Bog Snorkelling Championships when we came close to Builth Wells, and yes you guessed it, Jack was insistent on joining

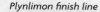

Plynlimon finish line

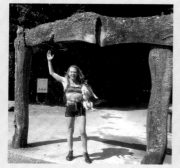

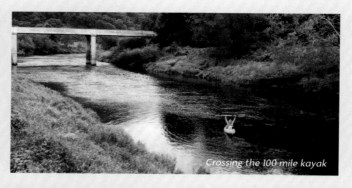

Crossing the 100 mile kayak

me in the bog for this mucky fun-swim. The organisers were so welcoming to my little Jack and his wild Mum, who had caused a proper stir on their recent adventure.

Jack was always a welcome sight, greeting me at my many pit stops during my river swim and we were quickly coming to the last few days of our Wye-cation. It was sad in some ways, but had been so much fun and we had made and 'banked' another totally wonderful memory that neither of us will ever forget.

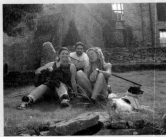

BBC documentary

The BBC followed us on some sections of our adventure, as they wanted to document our connection to the wildlife in our natural office and playground. I only agreed to be part of the BBC documentary if they showed how wonderful the great outdoors is and how Jack and I really loved and appreciated the lifestyle it gave us.

Admittedly, it did get rather frustrating sometimes, trying to be free whilst being filmed but luckily the crew only caught up with us every five or six days, which meant we had lots of 'free-time' in between. And the outcome was a wonderful film, documenting one of my and Jack's adventures on the Wye side. And of course we kept our amusement to ourselves.

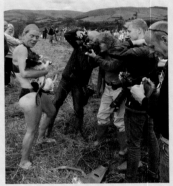

World bog snorkelling

And finally when our documentary comes out on the BBC Jack falls asleep watching himself on his adventures.

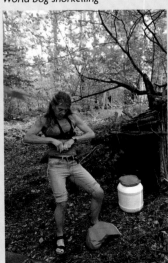

Supplies hidden along the Wye

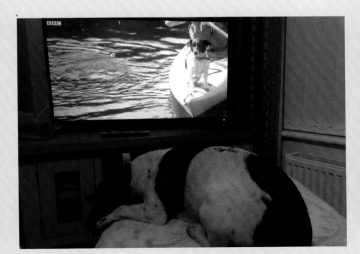

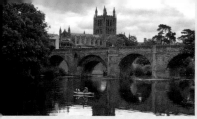
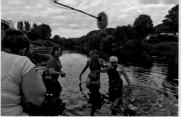
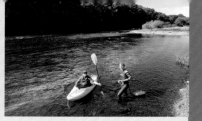

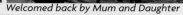
Welcomed back by Mum and Daughter

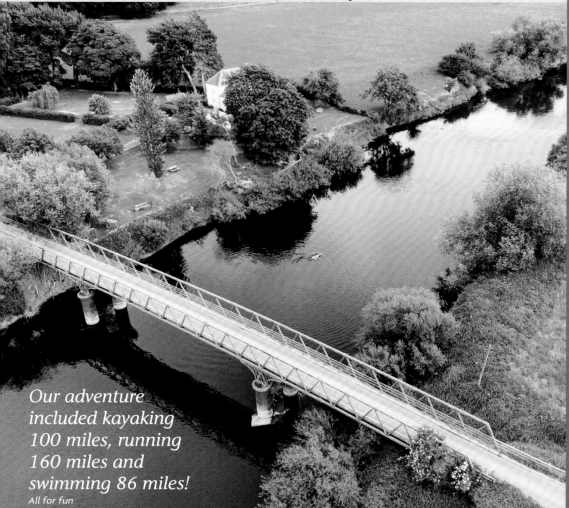

Our adventure included kayaking 100 miles, running 160 miles and swimming 86 miles!
All for fun

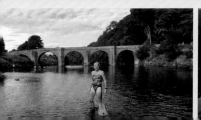
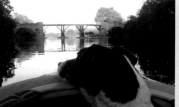
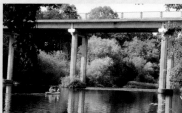

World Bog Snorkelling Champs

Jack and I have done many spontaneous fun things in our lives and this was no different as we were on a busman's holiday for 5 weeks. Running, kayaking, swimming and sleeping out on the River Wye, we popped over to do the World Bog Snorkelling Championships (which I've done many times before for charities and purely for fun).

This time, Jack insisted he joined me. He screeched with excitement at the first sight of water, and was adamant he joined me for the whole swim. Laughed, we were ecstatic and so pleased that the organisers allowed my Jack to be the first little doggy to join his pet parent in the water. We never apply pressure to do times or distances, just good old fun!

And we so love the earthy peat of our glorious Welsh hills and the rich peat bogs.

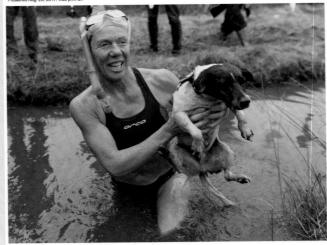

NEW YORK POST

Underwater with the World Bog Snorkelling Championship 2017

By Emil Lendof
Published Aug. 28, 2017, 4:38 p.m. ET

LLANWRTYD WELLS, WALES -- AUGUST 27: Angela Jones exits the water with her dog Jack who also completed the swim during the World Bog Snorkelling Championships 2017 on August 27,....

Getty Images

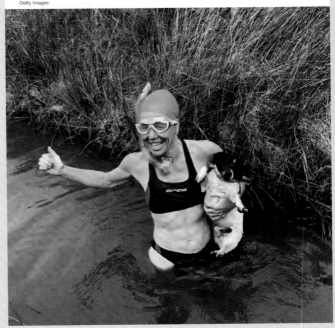

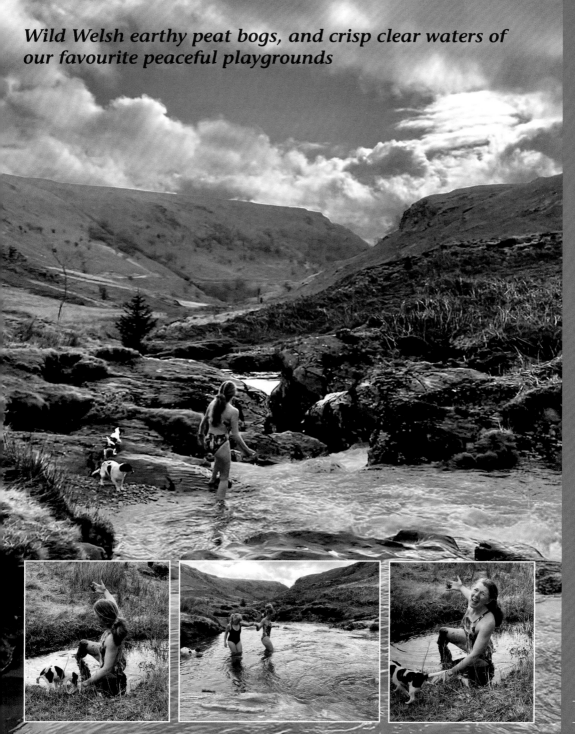

Wild Welsh earthy peat bogs, and crisp clear waters of our favourite peaceful playgrounds

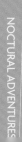

Early sunrise over the Wye, towards Lydbrook

Image: M. Gray

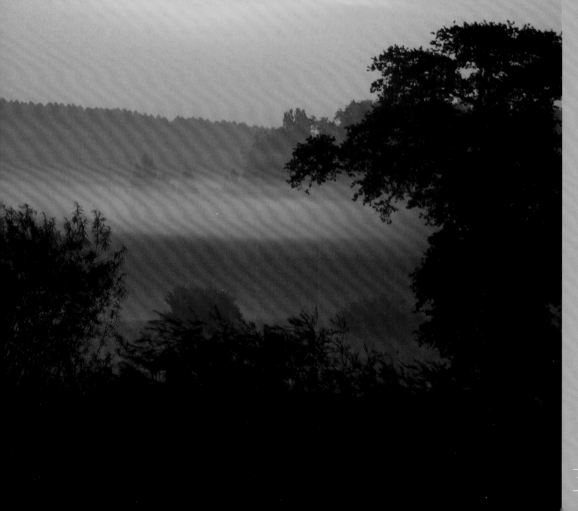

"The earth doesn't belong to us,
we belong to the earth.

What we do to the earth
we do to ourselves."

CHIEF SEATTLE

Nocturnal Adventures in Nature

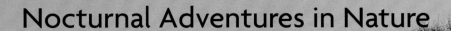

Our days of 'wild wandering' overlap into 'evocative evenings', where our enjoyment of nocturnal Nature comes alive, especially when swimming, which offers the unbridled privilege of sharing the watery space with Nature in the twilight. It sharpens your senses beautifully and simply makes your soul soar.

I adore exploring and discovering a wild world that is not often seen, but which is a definite favourite of mine and Jack's.

Often we combine a night swim with wild camping on the river's edge, where Nature puts on such a special show, and often offers us glimpses of something special. Jack has been brought up with a serenity that allows him to watch and absorb his surroundings and the wonderful wildlife, without any thought for chasing or barking. We make a tight team,

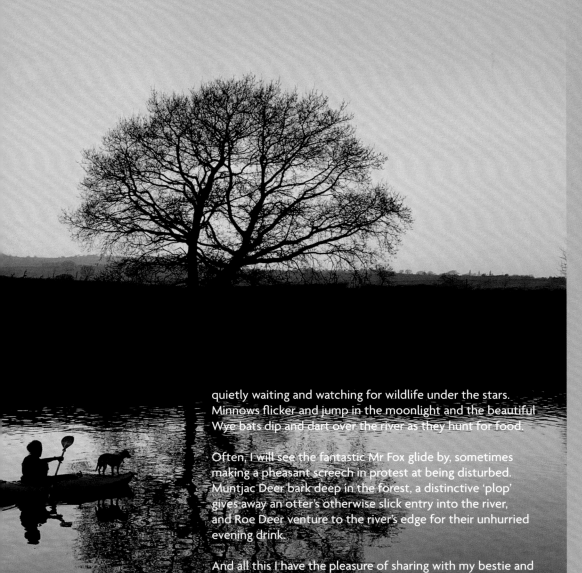

quietly waiting and watching for wildlife under the stars. Minnows flicker and jump in the moonlight and the beautiful Wye bats dip and dart over the river as they hunt for food.

Often, I will see the fantastic Mr Fox glide by, sometimes making a pheasant screech in protest at being disturbed. Muntjac Deer bark deep in the forest, a distinctive 'plop' gives away an otter's otherwise slick entry into the river, and Roe Deer venture to the river's edge for their unhurried evening drink.

And all this I have the pleasure of sharing with my bestie and my woof, Jack.

Far from provoking fear, the dark provides another, different kind of magical show for us from Nature – and it is always an absolute privilege to be in the audience.

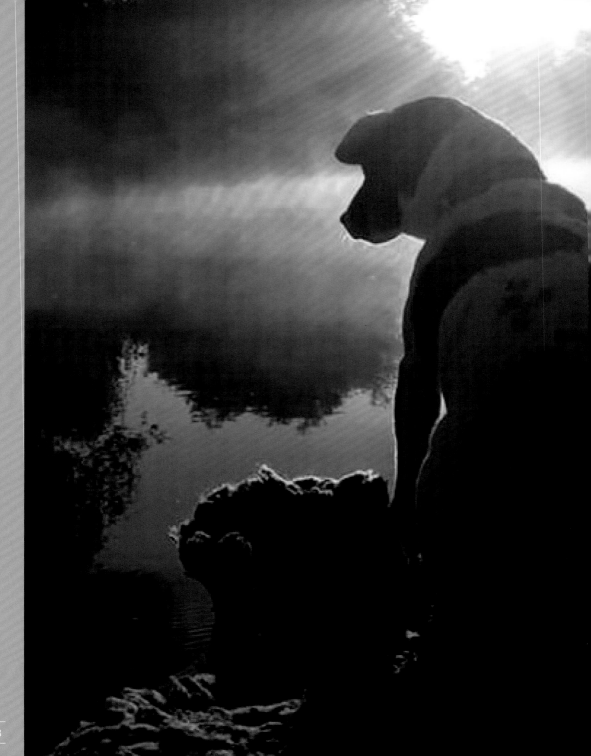

> *"Far from provoking fear, the dark provides another magical show from Nature – and it is an absolute privilege to be in the audience."*

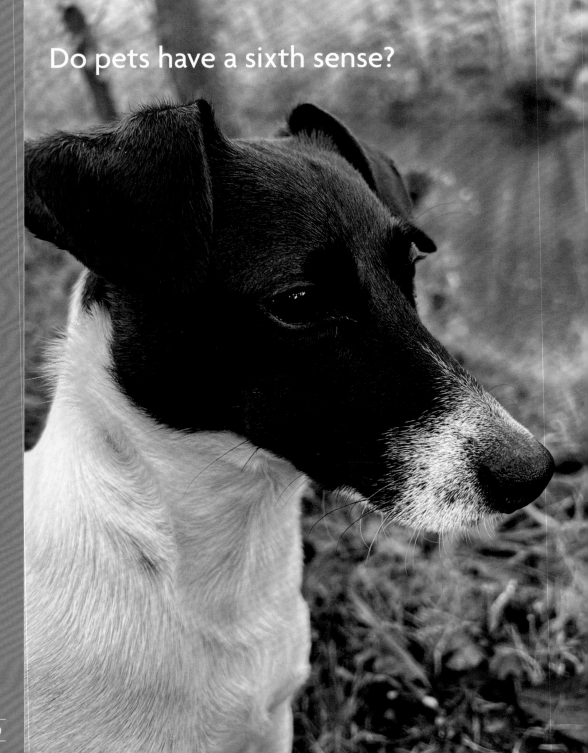

Do pets have a sixth sense?

Senses

Humans have five recognised senses. We taste, touch, smell, see, and hear. Likewise, dogs have the same five senses, but many people, including myself, think that dogs have 'one up on us'.

Canine Senses

Although dogs and humans have the same five senses, they aren't all exactly alike. When it comes to vision, humans have more colour detecting cells (cones) in the eye. These allow us to discern a broader colour spectrum and also allow us to detect more visual detail.

Sight

Dogs see better in the dark than humans. Canines have larger pupils that let in more light. Canine eyes also have more light sensitive cells (rods) in the centre of the retina. Both of these adaptations mean better vision in dim light. In addition, the canine eye detects tiny movements that may elude us. The canine sense of sight makes them good hunters, especially at night.

Smell

When it comes to smell, a dog's nose functions around 10,000 times better than ours, but our sense of taste beats theirs. Humans have about 9000 taste buds as compared to just around 1700 for dogs.

Hearing

Hearing is comparable, too, with regard to quality of sound. But dogs can detect much higher frequencies and can hear at much longer distances than we can.

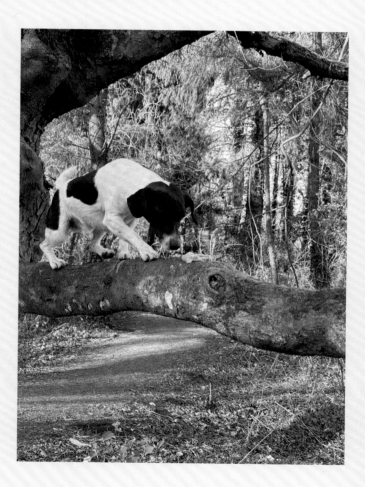

Sixth sense?

Like humans, dogs have five remarkably good senses, but do they have an elusive sixth sense? And what is a sixth sense, anyway? Can it really be defined?

Think of a sixth sense as intuition or a "gut feeling". The five recognised senses each give us fragments of information about our environment or circumstances, whereas a sixth sense draws from the cumulative information gathered by the other five senses and in doing so, can raise the level of awareness.

So is it an additional sense or a heightened appreciation of the other five senses?

Who knows? But it certainly contributes to the magical gift of being a pet parent – or a 'pawrent'.

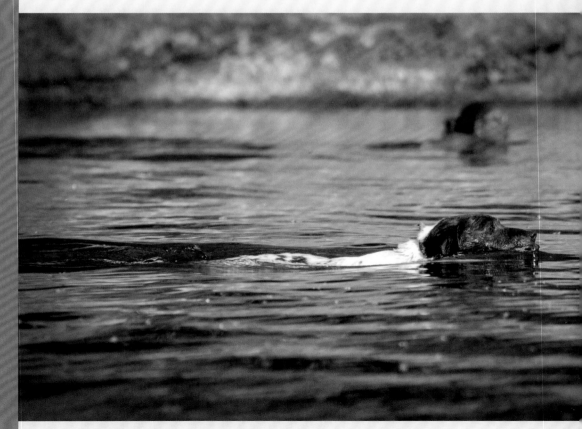

Jack would always sense a nervous client and would swim close to them to reassure them.

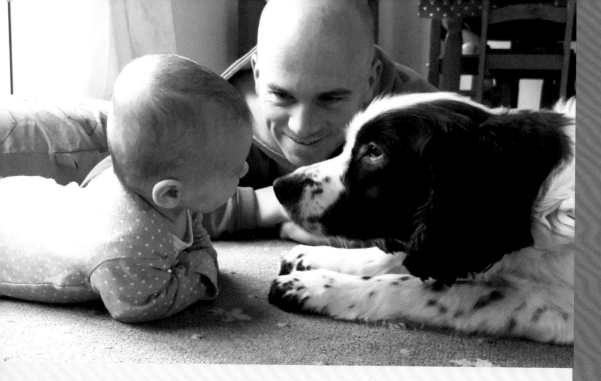

Sensitive Examples

Human Moods

Many pet parents know that their dogs are quite intuitive. When we are happy, our dogs may be equally exuberant, enjoying our happiness. When I'm excited – which is my default setting – my dogs have always mirrored my enthusiasm and zest for life.

Dogs will pick up on a sad or low mood and try to offer comfort by snuggling in or just giving us that understanding look.

Humans produce a group of 'feel good' hormones, such as oxytocin, serotonin, and dopamine. The levels of these hormones increase and decrease along with the elevation or depression of our moods. When we are sick, our dogs may detect a fall in hormone levels and respond accordingly. As they comfort us, hormone levels may rise and we feel better. How rewarding for our dogs when they detect this rise and realise that their presence helped us feel better!

So our furry friends seem to know what we need; but how? Is it our facial expressions or our voice or our body language, or our hormones or our smell? Or is it that 'sixth sense'?

I can't tell you how many times this came into play with my beloved Jack over the years – the examples are simply endless.

Dogs have an acute sense of hearing, and will hear distant thunder long before we do. They also smell changes in the atmosphere (ozone) better than we do, so they may sense an oncoming storm. When my Jack got anxious I knew there was going to be a change in the weather. Jack was my own little 'weather forecaster', 100% more reliable than any tech or phone apps and extremely helpful for our adventures.

Two thirds of pet owners think their pets have a sixth sense about weather – and we should be very appreciative of them sharing that gift with us. It is not just about whether or not we should 'take a coat' but there are many safety connotations attached to being able to predict unfavourable weather conditions, especially when out on rural adventures. Of course, this only works if we 'take notice'.

A dog's keen sense of smell can also enable them to "sense" some human illnesses. When we are sick, our body chemistry changes, giving off a scent that is only picked up by our furry friends.

Dogs quickly learn the routines of the people they live with, but Jack had the added ability to know that every day was going to be adventurous and an unpredictable one. He learned that there were 'no dramas', life was good and all was well – this enabled him to be chilled and stress-free.

How can you sense your pet's sixth sense?

We may not be as sensitive as our dogs, but we all recognise when a dog's sixth sense is 'switched on.' They may bark. They may seek out their owners. They may be agitated or anxious. You (should) know your pet and they will (definitely) know you. Just pay attention and you may be surprised at how intuitive they are. And even though there is no scientific evidence regarding a dog's sixth sense, we certainly have "sense" enough to appreciate our dogs' awesome abilities and how they integrate their other five senses in an amazing fashion.

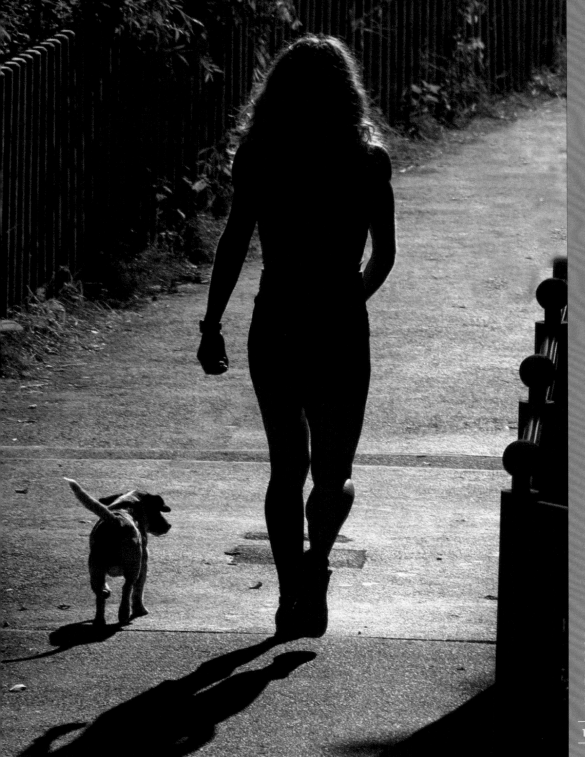

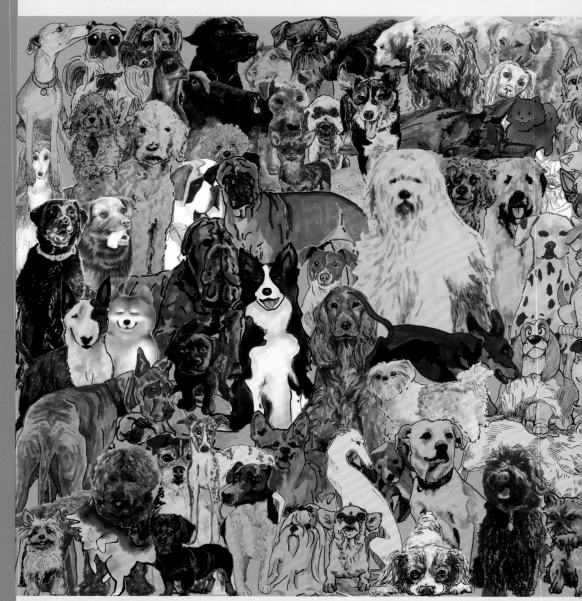

Over 900 million dogs in the world; many wild but all wonderful

Endorsements:

Lynne Albutt - *Writer, TV presenter*
Angela's latest book, following on from the success of '***Wild Swimming the River Wye***', continues to chronicle her love, respect and passion for the great outdoors, whilst sharing more 'wild skills', inspiring stories and essential safety advice to enable you to include your canine companion in all of your outdoor adventures safely and with regard for nature and wildlife.

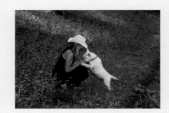

Mrs Jean Mary Morris *BVSc MRCVS.*
A well-respected vet of 60 years.
This book is full of good down to earth advice on how we and our canine friends can enjoy safely the great outdoors and its surroundings without damaging the environment. Angela writes with such enthusiasm which is transferred to the reader. I admire all she does with such courage and determination, lets hope it has an impact on us all.

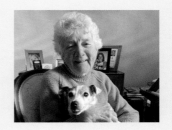

Dr David Lee - *Wildlife Ecologist and Conservation Scientist, Biologist and Explorer*
Angela's deep love of our countryside and engaging people with it is only matched by her indefatigable commitment to improving and protecting our glorious rivers. She is a force for positive change, and the world needs more Angelas.

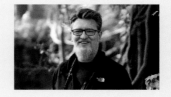

Kate Humble *BBC Wildlife & TV Presenter, Writer and Broadcaster*
Angela Jones is the most energetic and impassioned protector and champion of our countryside I know. She, and her ever faithful four-pawed companion Jack, are the best guides you could possibly want to help you enjoy and appreciate this beautiful country.

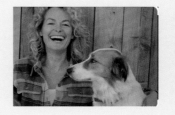

James Smith - *Highly acclaimed BBC Wildlife Producer and BAFTA Winner. BAFTA-winning producer for the Amazon and Arctic series. He has lead expeditions in the Congo Basin and Alaska for BBC1 and Discovery. Producer for Spring, Autumn, Winter Watch and Wild Wales*
An Inspiring book about sharing wild adventures with your dog and the connection with Nature, written with true heart by the remarkable Wild Wye Woman.

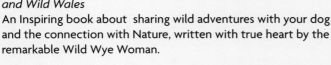

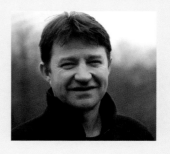

Wild adventures with your canine friend

Author: Angela Jones - www.angelajonesswimwild.co.uk

Editing;   Lynn Allbutt and David Evans

Design & Layout: Sherren McCabe-Finlayson - Platform One: www.platform-one.co.uk

Proceeds from this book will go to: Helping my Environmental Campaign to protect our rivers, Canine Rescue and our local Children's Hospice as Jack so adored children.

Acknowledgements

My second book has been 2 years in the making and something I passionately wanted to persevere to complete. It means so much to me and is a tribute to my best friend, adventurer and soul-mate for 14 years; my dear Jack Russell "Jack".

Once again, as I mention in my first book, being Dyslexic, never being able to read a book and having no home internet makes it not an easy task. This book has very much been a challenge and has been achieved the good old-fashioned way – hard work and battling on. I have had great pleasure in accomplishing and it gives me joy to share what truly means so much to me and Jack, while hopefully inspiring others to respect and protect our great outdoors with their four-legged friends.

A lifetime in Nature on the wildside has taught me plenty, and to transfer my immense knowledge and safety skills with others has been a true pleasure and, very importantly, keeping my canine friends safe.

11 million dogs in the UK and so many Pet parents taking to new adventures is also a reason to write this book.

Thank you so much to all who have contributed to our book :

Lynne Allbutt

This could not be possible without the fantastic support in editing from a kindred spirit in Mother Nature, Lynne Allbutt. This amazing lady has been so unfazed and generous with her time and abundance of clever editing skills. She truly connects with the love of being a pet parent and with the great outdoors.

Stuart Pearce

Has been once again a great part of my second book as of my first; by structure, editorial, and capturing some amazing photos of me and Jack over the years. And of course a great sounding board !!

Platform One

A big shout out to Sher and David from Platform one for putting my book together so beautifully and skilfully. You have been so supportive and helped me share my vision by bringing my book to life in exactly the way I wanted !! Your friendship and professionalism is gratefully appreciated.

Nicola Turner

Nicola and her canine pet Pixel have appeared in this book. Nick Demonstrates and writes about her knowledge of core training skills and culinary healthy doggy snacks. Nick has been a true supporter and friend and a wonderful addition to this book .

Michelle Flight

Michelle's stunning photographs of her spaniel wonder dog Willow have appeared throughout the book; also some amazing landscape photographs. Once again, being part of both my books she shares her love of the outdoors through her amazing art of photography .

Gemma Katewood

Gemma's wonderful photographs play a beautiful part in capturing my and Jack's love of the outdoors. Thank you for sharing so generously.

Jean Morris

What a wonderful privilege to share time with such an inspirational warm-hearted person. Your love and knowledge for the animal world as a vet is second to none. You welcomed me from day one and allowed me to ask many questions and gather much information. Your many decades as a Vet and your beautiful caring nature is truly admired. Thank you.

Laura Eden Artist

Laura has contributed to much artwork through this book, from illustrations to her own beautiful pieces, and also sharing her students' work on this project. She has not faltered on the constant amount of work I've put her way! A true friend and a beautiful Pet Parent.

Beautifully painted illustrations which are a privilege to show. Page 157

Finally, to all the wonderful Adventure clients over the years who have joined me and Jack on the Wildside. Thank you for allowing me to use your photos and being part of our Wild Journey.

Laura Eden, Willow Harper, Rebecca Martin, Maia Lewis, Bethan Roberts, Lillie Coop, Liwsi Cowin, Eva Smets, Sienna Lewis, Elis Marriott, Betty Angell, Cameron Breese. A collaboration of artists from across Cardiff, Monmouth, Chippenham and Taunton.

Photo Contributors

Jill Berryman, Jane Mansfield, Grey family, Daniela Gormley, Jan Richards, Michelle Flight, Arunn Jones, Kayla Methuen, Bronwen Morgan, Iain MacDonald, Nic Turner, Stuart Pearce, Gemma Katewood, Dinsdale family.

Safe paddling, Dogs Senses, Health tips have been used for research.

Published May 2024

The moral right of Angela Jones to be identified as the author of this work has been asserted in accordance with the Copyright, Designs and Patents Act of 1998.

ISBN: 978-1-8380857-2-8

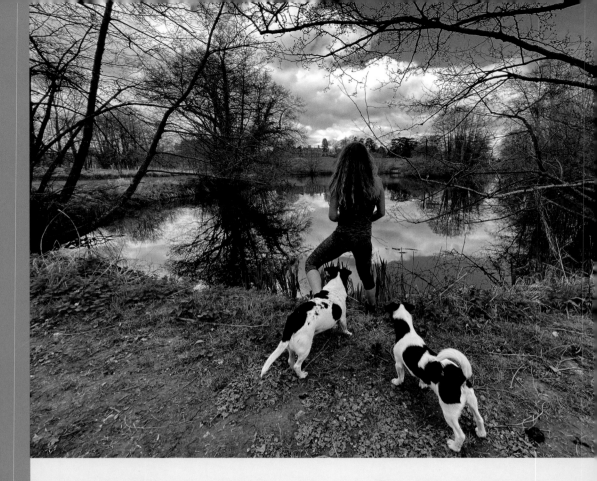

My Adventurer and best friend Jack

We are going on one last journey along the Wye from Source to Sea – 155 miles.

Celebrating an amazing 14 years of fun and adventures together; doing some kayaking, swimming and wild camping – everything we both loved, but at a slower relaxed pace: Jack pace.

To celebrate Jack's life we will be doing this for the local Children's Hospice I'm ambassador for, as Jack adored children and their laughter, and what better way to celebrate his life but to give back to those that need it?

Being with him for 14 years on the Wildside it is difficult to say goodbye, but my life, like Jack's has always been about the positives, the here and now, the fun, the adventures, the love of embracing every minute of it!
And now over to Junior.